ABOUT THE AUTHORS

EMBREE DE PERSIIS VONA, a graduate of McGill University, is a professional pot-
ter who lives in Big Sur, California. She developed her enthusiasm for health food
in the mid '60s, "when [she] started feeding [herself]."

ANSTICE CARROLL lives in New York City, where she has owned and run the
Anstice Carroll Catering Company for 25 years, and where she was food direc-
tor at the Grace Church School in Greenwich Village for 27 years.

GIANNA DE PERSIIS VONA became obsessed with health food after the birth of
her two sons. Besides being knowledgeable in the realm of health food and natural healing, Gianna is a cook and a writer. She has a Masters Degree in creative
writing and leads inspirational writing workshops in her hometown of
Sebastopol, California. Her advice column "Ask Sydney" appears weekly in
Women's Voices, and on-line at www.asksydney.com.

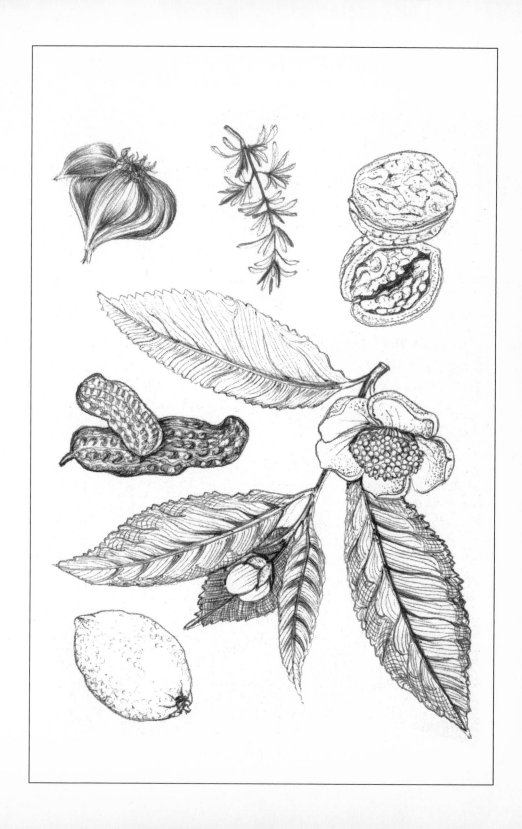

THE
DICTIONARY
OF
WHOLESOME
FOODS

A PASSIONATE A-TO-Z GUIDE TO THE EARTH'S

HEALTHY OFFERINGS, WITH MORE THAN

140 DELICIOUS, NUTRITIOUS RECIPES

Anstice Carroll, Embree De Persiis Vona,
and Gianna De Persiis Vona

Illustrated by Vincenzo De Persiis Vona

MARLOWE & COMPANY
NEW YORK

THE DICTIONARY OF WHOLESOME FOODS:
*A Passionate A-to-Z Guide to the Earth's Healthy Offerings,
with More than 140 Delicious, Nutritious Recipes*

Copyright © 2006 by Anstice Carroll, Embree De Persiis Vona, and Gianna De Persiis Vona

This is a revised, updated, and expanded edition
of *The Health Food Dictionary*, originally published by
Prentice-Hall International, Inc., in 1973.
© 1973 by Anstice Carroll and Embree De Persiis Vona

Illustrations by Vincenzo De Persiis Vona

Published by
Marlowe & Company
An Imprint of Avalon Publishing Group Incorporated
245 West 17th Street • 11th floor
New York, NY 10011–5300

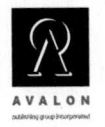

AVALON
publishing group incorporated

Library of Congress Cataloging-in-Publication Data
Carroll, Anstice.
[Health food dictionary with recipes]
The dictionary of wholesome foods : a passionate A-to-Z guide to the earth's healthy offerings, with more than 140 delicious, nutritious recipes / by Anstice Carroll, Embree De Persiis Vona, and Gianna De Persiis Vona ; illustrations by Vicenzo De Persiis Vona.
p. cm.
"Originally published as The Health Food Dictionary
by Prentice-Hall International, Inc., in 1973."
ISBN: 1-56924-395-6
1. Food—Dictionaries. 2. Cookery—Dictionaries.
I. De Persiis Vona, Embree, 1941- II. De Persiis Vona, Gianna. III. Title.
TX349.C39 2006
641.303—dc22   2005031151

ISBN-13: 978-1-56924-395-4

9 8 7 6 5 4 3 2 1

Designed by Pauline Neuwirth, Neuwirth and Associates

Printed in the United States of America

For my daughter Brynne, and for my mother and father
A. C. C.

❧

For my son and daughter, Pietro and Gianna
E. D. P. V.

❧

For my mother, Embree, who raised me on the
original version of this book
G. D. P. V.

❧

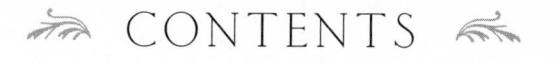

CONTENTS

THE DICTIONARY OF WHOLESOME FOODS

❧ PREFACE ❧

WHEN *The Health Food Dictionary,* as it was then aptly penned, was originally written, Anstice Carroll and Embree De Persiis Vona were pioneers in a field of their own invention, health food for the gourmet inclined. Sure, they wanted to be healthy, to raise their children on wholesome foods, and the purest ingredients whenever possible, but they weren't about to give up their double espressos with organic milk or the butter on their thick slices of homemade bread. They sought to demystify health food, to identify it, and in so doing to make it both more accessible and tempting to the layperson and health food addict alike. Some thirty years later, the majority of the original book has held the test of time. Certainly a few things have been changed, but the changes are slight enough as to be almost unnoticeable. There was no need. The previous *Health Food Dictionary* was so comprehensive and insightful that I still use my original copy, published in 1973, with such frequency that it is egg-spattered, flour-coated, and generally in such miserable condition that it is abundantly clear that not only do I love it, but I do not take very good care of my cookbooks. Even the family heirlooms.

It has been a great privilege for me to be involved in the "second coming" of what has always held a certain mystique in my family—my mother, Embree, and Anstice's dictionary and recipe book, with intricately designed illustrations by my late father, Vincenzo. Though the book went through seven printings, original copies are scarce and therefore coveted. My best friend attempted to get ahold of my copy for years, many a time trying to guilt me into giving it to her, and when my mother finally located one at a used book store and gave it to her as a gift, I was just a little bit jealous. The fact that both Embree and Anstice have welcomed me into the dictionary lineage has been an honor for me, and I set about discovering new ingredients and putting them here, along with an array of fantastic new recipes, mostly provided by Anstice Carroll, caterer extraordinaire. Between the three of us—Anstice's recipes, Embree's outstanding writing and editing skills, and my willingness to perform the information sleuthing the second time around—we have made something new, *The Dictionary of Wholesome Foods,* which is the original with a much-needed and long-time-coming modern twist. While many new entries have been added, such as amaranth and kombucha, as well as recipes for Tuscan marinade, and chickpea with basmati rice salad, among others, the simple and accessible structure remains the same, and in a time where pesticide-laden and preservative-rich foods drown the market, and threats of genetically modified foods loom on the horizon and begin to infiltrate our grocery stores, it is never too late to pick up this book and begin to understand some simple ways of adding a little wholesome zest to your everyday diet.

—Gianna De Persiis Vona, *October 2005*

A WARNING

This book is *not* for the health food fanatic!

A STATEMENT OF INTENT

This book is for the person who browses through a health food store—be it for the first or the hundredth time—and feels overwhelmed or at least slightly confused. And it is also for gourmets who have no intention whatsoever of giving up their croissants and espresso in favor of brewer's yeast or blackstrap molasses, but who would like to *gently ease* a little more health into their lives.

You do not have to completely change your lifestyle, become a bore on the subject, stop going out to dinner, or drop your unhealthy friends in order to reap the benefits of a more organic way of life. With only a few changes, and delicious ones at that, you can fulfill your wish to eat healthfully and still have delicious food at every meal.

SOME PROBLEMS

The health food field is burgeoning, becoming more intricate, and many questions arise. Just what is an organic vegetable—how is it better than its sprayed counterpart; does it taste better; why does it cost more; how can you be sure it's organic; what if it is organic but just doesn't taste as good as what you get at the supermarket? What to do with all those flours—stone ground, pneumatically ground; hard wheat, soft wheat; graham flour, pastry flour—what are the differences between them; what's best for what; can you turn out bread with them that will satisfy your Italian mother-in-law as well as your macrobiotic nephew? Why buy raw milk when your grandmother remembers children dying from unpasteurized milk; can certified raw milk be trusted? What is an organic vitamin; why is it more expensive than its chemical counterpart? What are organic cosmetics; how can you know they are really better than the usual ones when the labels do not tell you what is in them?

How to answer all the questions? First read this book; you will be placing your feet on firm ground. Then case the local health food outlets. Critically. Ask questions and do not be intimidated by eclectic atmospheres—health food should be for everybody, not just the chosen few. Use this book as a dictionary—to clarify, to verify, to raise questions about what you have seen. Ask where the store gets its vegetables, dried fruits, and nuts. Ask if they have been tested for insecticide residues. Visit the farm sources if they are local and you are keen. Your aim is good, healthful, uncontaminated food. Demand it!

AND WE ALSO HAVE RECIPES

Now supposing you have found a good dependable health food store. You buy a little whole wheat flour, a little honey, maybe a few nuts. You buy one of the doctrinaire health food cookbooks off the rack. You get home, decide to cook up something healthy, look it up in the book—cookies maybe—and by gosh but aren't there ten ingredients in those almond cookies that you don't have in the kitchen! What to do? Go back to the store and spend a small fortune buying all that strange stuff just to cook up one batch of cookies? *Don't do it!* For here, in this dictionary, you will find simple recipes based on only one or two health food items apiece—the rest of the ingredients you can scrounge out of the most ordinary kitchen (of course, the healthier the better). We will also tell you how to make do with whole wheat flour when a recipe calls for pastry flour; how to substitute honey for sugar and vice versa; how to make flaxseed meal when all you have in the cupboard is flaxseed; and other helpful hints.

Additional feature: cut down on your stockpile of aspirin and tranquilizers by following our herbal tea hints. Don't believe it? Try it.

Happy reading, shopping, cooking, and eating to you, in the name of health and common sense.

—The Authors

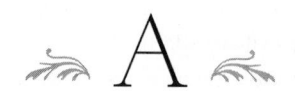

A

ACEROLA CHERRY   The acerola cherry, also called Barbados cherry, is a tropical fruit known for its high vitamin C content. In appearance it resembles the common American cherry, but botanically the two are not related. Fantastic claims are made for its vitamin C qualities—some scientists maintain that 6 ounces of acerola cherries yield as much of the precious vitamin as 50 pounds of fresh cabbage juice (cabbage itself is known for its high vitamin C content). At any rate, that this cherry is far higher in natural vitamin C than any other known food is indisputable.

Acerola cherries are often combined with rose hips in vitamin C pills and liquid drops (these are very convenient for infants and young children—and the taste is naturally agreeable).

ACIDOPHILUS MILK   This is a cultured milk into which acidophilus bacteria have been introduced. It is not a very stable product and must be used within a couple of days of the making. Therefore it is rarely sold commercially. Acidophilus milk aids the growth of healthful intestinal flora and at the same time inhibits the growth of unfriendly bacteria—in much the same manner as yogurt, except that the acidophilus is far stronger (and, incidentally, not so appetizing).

In health food stores you will find liquid acidophilus culture and acidophilus food powder. The liquid culture is taken by the teaspoonful or mixed with water or juice. Acidophilus "food" may be taken in conjunction with the culture and feeds the acidophilus bacteria, making them work more ambitiously. The culture is also available in pill form.

ADZUKI BEAN   This small, dark red bean looks almost too good to eat, more like a polished stone to be treasured than to be treated as a mere dried bean.

Dark red is how we usually see it, though straw-colored, brown, and even black adzuki beans are also to be found.

The adzuki is native to Japan, where it is valued highly for its vitamin and mineral content. Those who follow a macrobiotic regimen use it in an endless variety of ways—alone as a vegetable, mixed with rice or other grains, even as pie filling. The juice derived by boiling the adzuki is said to be beneficial to the kidneys.

Adzuki are delicious as a substitute for black-eyed peas in that mainstay of Southern dishes, Hoppin' John. The result is rather more delicate than the original and truly fit for a gourmet's table.

ADZUKI RICE

½ cup adzuki beans

3 cups water

1½ teaspoons salt

½ cup brown rice

1 tablespoon butter

- Soak adzuki beans in 1 cup water for 2 hours. Then cook slowly in the same liquid for about 1 hour, until slightly tender.
- Bring 2 cups water to a boil. Add salt. Sprinkle rice into water without disturbing boiling. Add adzuki beans and their liquid. Cover and cook slowly for 45 minutes. Add butter.
- This side dish is also good when served cold. Toss with a little olive oil and garnish with chopped fresh herbs.
- Serves four.
- *Note:* If shorter-cooking rice is used, cook the adzuki beans 30 minutes longer before adding to rice.

AGAR-AGAR   Agar-agar, sometimes called Japanese or vegetable gelatin (or just plain agar), comes from a type of seaweed. It is widely used as a thickener and emulsifier by the food processing industry (and among its many other uses finds great service in laboratories as a culture medium). Vegetarians use it to replace common gelatin, which is made from animal protein.

Agar-agar will jell salads and dessert gelatins and thicken soups. When agar-agar is used, fruit and vegetable juices can be jelled merely by warming rather than by boiling, and therefore more of their health value is retained. Jellies and jams made with agar-agar rather than commercial pectin do not need nearly as much sugar or honey (pectin products are very sour, and the large amounts of sugar called for are needed more to compensate for this sourness than for that of the fruit). Agar-agar is also useful in cases of constipation, for it swells to many times its bulk when it reaches the intestines and increases peristaltic action without causing painful griping

Agar-agar comes in flake, granulated, and bar form. These are the basic proportions to use: 3½ cups liquid to 2 tablespoons flakes; 3½ cups liquid to 1 tablespoon granulated; 3½ cups liquid to approximately 7 inches bar form. In all instances, soak the agar-agar in 1 cup of liquid for 10 minutes, then warm on stove until dissolved; add rest of liquid, which should be at room temperature. Refrigerate if desired, but this will jell without refrigeration.

AGAVE NECTAR (*uh-gah-vay*) Extracted from the pineapple-shaped core of the agave, a cactuslike plant, the agave was traditionally cultivated in the hills of Mexico. The ancients considered the agave to be a sacred plant with properties to purify the body and soul. The Spaniards, who apparently had their own ideas with regard to self-purification, took this same juice, fermented it, and created what we now call tequila.

Agave syrup, or nectar (it's the same thing), is 90 percent fruit sugar and has a consistency similar to that of honey. Sweeter than sugar, less is needed for any recipe—¾ cups agave nectar is equal to 1 cup of sugar. Be sure to reduce the liquid in recipes by almost one-half when using agave in place of sugar.

AJOWAN Native to India, ajowan seeds, which are similar in appearance to celery seeds, have a pungent, thymelike flavor and scent. Commonly used in Indian lentil dishes and bread, ajowan should be used sparingly, as its flavor is strong.

When smoked, the seeds are said to relieve asthma. Essential oil of ajowan is used as an antiseptic and carminative.

ALFALFA The benefits to be derived from this "animal food" should be given their due. Alfalfa is a leguminous plant that has been cultivated for over two thousand years as forage; horses have waxed swift and strong on its healthful properties—and so well might you. The roots of the alfalfa grow extraordinarily deep into the earth and are able to probe out minerals and trace elements that more shallow-rooted plants cannot reach. Alfalfa is also a rich source of vitamins and contains all eight essential amino acids, calcium, phosphorus, potassium, and iron. Its richness in vitamin A makes it a particularly good food for pregnant and nursing women, and it is said to increase the flow of breast milk. It is helpful in cleansing toxins from the bloodstream, fighting infections in the body, hindering tooth decay, treating anemia, healing ulcers, and boosting the immune system.

Chew the leaves raw, add them to salad, or sauté them in oil and serve as a tender vegetable.

Alfalfa is available in health food stores in pill, powder, tea, and seed (for sprouting) form.

ALFALFA LEAF TEA   This tea, in addition to its superior nutritive values (see *Alfalfa*), is very easily assimilated and therefore particularly good for the elderly and for children. Its rather bland flavor becomes extremely tasty when mixed with mint. To brew alfalfa tea, steep 1 teaspoon alfalfa leaves in 2 cups boiling water for about 10 minutes.

ALFALFA POWDER   Alfalfa leaves can be finely ground into a flourlike powder, which is used as a food supplement. It can be added to a glass of juice or to your bread (½ cup alfalfa powder to 5 cups flour), soups, and stews. Keep in mind, however, that some hay fever sufferers turn out to be allergic to alfalfa hay dust. See also *Alfalfa*.

ALFALFA SEED   These tiny seeds produce the tenderest and sweetest of sprouts (see *Sprouts* for simple growing instructions). Alfalfa sprouts are a perfect addition to sandwiches, for they will not go limp after a few hours like lettuce. Add them to salads or put a bowl of them on the table—you may find your children eating them by the handful, for they make an intriguing crunchy snack.

The seeds can be used, unsprouted, for tea—1 teaspoon seeds to 2 cups boiling water. The mild-tasting brew is said to be beneficial in cases of arthritis. See also *Alfalfa*.

ALLSPICE   True to its name, allspice tastes like cinnamon, nutmeg, and cloves all combined—if your taste buds can picture that! It is the hard berry of an evergreen tree native to the West Indies. The early Spanish explorers mistook this berry for the peppercorn, which it strongly resembles, and so it also came to be known as *pimienta* (Spanish for pepper) and Jamaican pepper. Its pungency enhances the flavor of mincemeat, pickles, and true Italian *mortadella* (a type of pork sausage). The whole berry can be used in marinades, pickles, or broths and gravies (strained). Ground allspice flavors curry and spicy cakes and cookies.

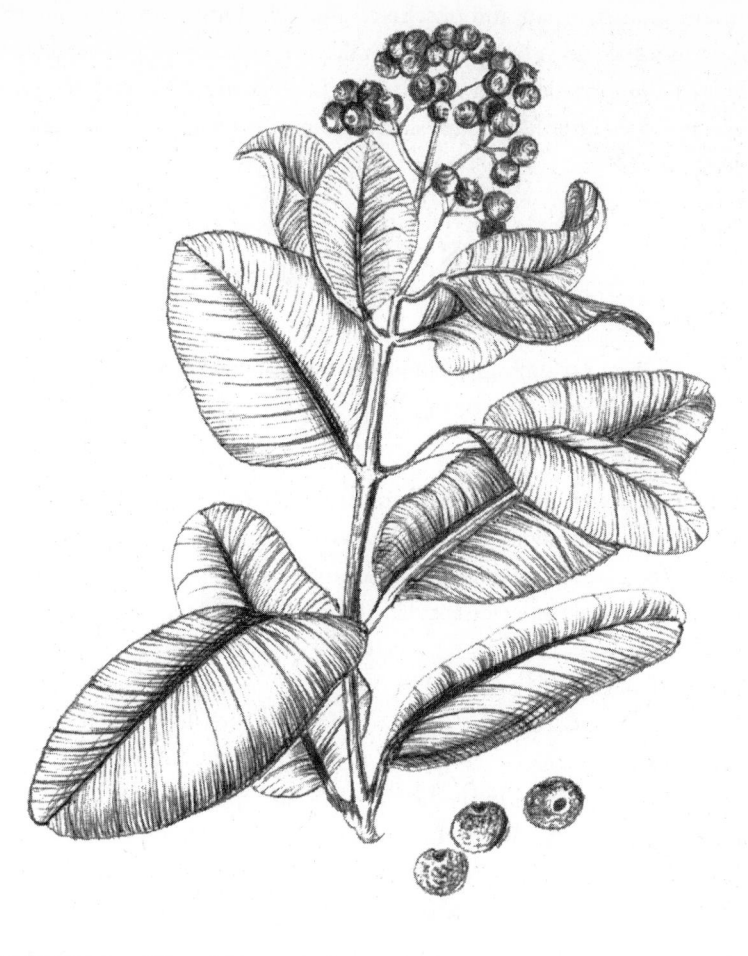

ALMOND   The edible seed of a peachlike tree, the almond is one of the most nutritious of nuts, containing large amounts of protein, vitamin B, calcium, potassium, magnesium, iron, and phosphorus. A few almonds go a long way—this is a highly concentrated food! As a meat substitute, almonds are very useful in vegetarian diets. The brown skin of the raw almond is sometimes irritating to the intestines, and it can be removed by blanching: pour boiling water over the nuts, let them sit for a minute, then slip off the skins—take care not to let the nuts get waterlogged. Ground blanched almonds are the essential ingredient of that European delicacy, marzipan. A milk made from crushed blanched almonds is sometimes recommended for stimulation of milk secretion in nursing mothers and as an easily digested healthful beverage for babies and children.

There are two varieties of almonds—sweet and bitter. The sweet nuts are the ones we enjoy for their flavor and nutritive value. The bitter almond is utterly unappealing in taste, and is poisonous as well, for it contains prussic acid (also known as hydrogen cyanide and HCN). The bitter almond is used to make almond extract for cooking and oil for skin use; refining removes all trace of poisonous elements.

❦ ALMOND CRESCENTS

1 cup (2 sticks) butter

3 tablespoons honey (or ½ cup raw sugar)

1 cup ground almonds (blanched or unblanched)

2 cups whole wheat pastry flour

1½ teaspoons vanilla

- Preheat the oven to 300 degrees. Butter cookie sheets.
- Cream butter. Add honey or sugar, almonds, flour, and vanilla. Mix well, flouring your hands to keep dough from sticking.
- Shape with fingers into crescent shapes and bake for 35 minutes on a greased cookie sheet.
- Makes 50 cookies.

ALMOND MILK　Used in medieval times, almond milk was a common ingredient for cooks. Useful during Lent, when the consumption of dairy products was forbidden to many on religious grounds, almond milk was also vital to the good cook due to the lack of refrigeration. Fresh cow milk was a luxury often not available to those who lived in the cities or lacked a cow, and many cooks depended on nuts (predominantly almonds), which could be ground, mixed with boiling water, and then poured through a sieve—a process that created a high-fat milk alternative that was easy to make and did not spoil on the shelves.

Almonds are naturally high in protein, vitamin E, and a variety of minerals, including zinc, potassium, magnesium, calcium, and iron. Almond milk can be used as a replacement for dairy milk in any recipe and yields a rich, sweet, nutty flavor to baked goods. See also *Almond*.

ALMOND OIL　Almond oil is widely used in making cosmetics. In its pure state it is a skin conditioner; it is also good for soothing sunburn and for use as a massage oil. See also *Almond*.

AMARANTH   Once fed to Aztec warriors and runners, this 8,000-year-old plant (which is actually a broadleaf plant, not a grain) sports beautiful flowers of purple, gold, orange, and red and was once widely cultivated by the Aztecs. Cortez, apparently unaware of the incredible health benefits of this protein and vitamin-rich plant, considered the Aztec worship of amaranth to be idolatry and ordered the fields burned and anyone who was found possessing it to be violently punished.

Organically grown and GMO-free (GMO is an abbreviation for "genetically modified organisms"), amaranth, which is native to India and the Americas, is rich in iron, protein, lysine, and calcium. Amaranth is reputed to be useful in the treatment of heavy menstrual bleeding.

Amaranth flour is gluten-free and can be added in small amounts to breads and baked goods for nutritional zeal. Amaranth leaves and stems are also edible and are considered by many to be a high delicacy. The fresh leaves can be sautéed or eaten raw in salads. The amaranth seeds can be popped like popcorn for a nutritional treat.

AMAZAKE   Enjoyed by the Japanese for hundreds of years, amazake is a naturally sweet drink made from *koji* (cultured rice). The koji is mixed with water and whole grain rice and incubated until the enzymes begin to break down the carbohydrates and natural sweetness develops.

Amazake is rich in health benefits derived from the koji, including enzymes, B vitamins, niacin, thiamin, essential amino acids, and energy-providing glucose. The live enzymes in this dessertlike drink are said to strengthen the digestive system.

ANISE SEED   The dainty anise plant produces seeds of a most pungent nature. Native to the Near East, from whence it spread to Europe and America, anise seed has for centuries been valued by the cake and cookie maker; Romans chased down their feasts with anise cakes that were purported to aid digestion. Besides its pleasant licorice flavor, anise seed tea (1 teaspoon seeds to 2 cups boiling water) claims medicinal qualities for itself as a carminative and a reliever of coughing and asthma. Oil of anise is commonly used commercially in cough medicines.

Useful for sweetening the breath, treating flatulence, and increasing mother's milk, anise seed can be ground and used as a tea or taken in tincture form. Anise seeds are the essential ingredient of the liqueur anisette, a few drops of which will lend an exotic flair to your demitasse of espresso.

Star anise is the seed of a magnolia-type tree found in southern China and, strangely enough, it yields an aroma and oil identical to that of the anise plant. Some connoisseurs claim, however, that the odor of star anise is the more pungent of the two. Certainly star anise is beautiful—the dried pod is shaped like a star, and each of its sections partially encloses one tiny seed. In Asia it is sometimes regarded as a good luck charm.

Should you have a yen to emulate the gourmets of ancient Rome, try these anise wafers as a fitting finish for a heavy dinner.

ANISE WAFERS

½ cup sugar (preferably raw sugar)

3 teaspoons anise seed

1 cup (2 sticks) butter

1 egg

2 tablespoons brandy (or lemon juice)

2 cups whole wheat flour

1 cup unbleached white flour

1 teaspoon baking powder

½ teaspoon salt

½ teaspoon ground cinnamon

- Preheat oven to 350 degrees. Oil cookie sheets.
- Put sugar and anise seed in a blender and grind to a powder. Cream sugar-anise powder with the butter. Beat in egg and brandy. Sift in flour, baking powder, salt, and cinnamon. Mix well. Shape into a ball, wrap in wax paper or plastic, and chill for 30 minutes.
- Roll out on a floured board to ⅛-inch thickness. Cut into shapes with cookie cutters. Place on an oiled cookie sheet and bake for 12 minutes, or until brown.
- Makes about 60 cookies.

APPLE, DRIED   The dried apple is moist and nonsticky—a neat snack for children. It is not a particularly low-calorie food; however, its calories will work for, not against, you, because dried apples contain many valuable nutrients including pectin.

Dried apples can be soaked in water overnight and substituted with fairly good results in recipes that call for fresh apples. Stewed with a little honey and lemon juice added, they rest on their own merits.

APRICOT, DRIED   The apricot tree first gave fruit in Armenia and the mountainous regions of Asia; now, several thousand years later, it is grown in temperate climates throughout the world. Its dried fruit is a valuable source of vitamin A and also contains healthy amounts of potassium, niacin, sodium, magnesium, and iron—a very useful item! If you stew apricots or soak them overnight, they act as a mild purgative.

Avoid dried apricots whose color is too brilliant—they have probably been treated with sulfur. Those of more muted tones may not be as eye-catching, but they are usually tastier and far more healthful.

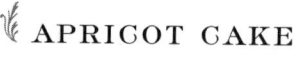 **APRICOT CAKE**

> 1 cup dried apricots (unsulfured)
>
> 1 cup water
>
> 2 cups sugar (preferably raw sugar)
>
> 10 tablespoons butter (1 stick plus 2 tablespoons)
>
> 1 teaspoon vanilla extract
>
> 1½ teaspoons lemon zest (organic undyed lemon, if possible)
>
> 2 eggs
>
> 2 cups whole wheat pastry flour, sifted
>
> ½ teaspoon salt
>
> 2¼ teaspoons baking powder
>
> 1 cup milk

Preheat oven to 350 degrees.

Soak apricots in water for about 2 hours. Place apricots and water, ½ cup sugar, and 2 tablespoons butter in a small saucepan over medium-low heat and simmer gently until sugar and butter dissolve. Purée mixture in a blender or food mill. Set aside.

Cream remaining butter and sugar. Add vanilla, lemon peel, and eggs one at a time, stirring well. Add flour, salt, and baking powder alternately with milk and beat until smooth, but do not overbeat.

Pour batter into an 8-inch buttered and floured springform pan. Spread apricot purée gently over top of batter, slightly thinner toward the middle. Bake at 350 degrees for about 1 hour, until cake pulls away from sides of pan. During baking, the apricot purée will penetrate the cake and end up in a layer at the bottom.

Top each piece with a dollop of whipped cream, or leave as is—delicious either way.

APRICOT KERNEL OIL This oil is used primarily as a cosmetic item. The hundred-year-old ladies of Hunza, Pakistan, are said to owe their wrinkle-free complexions to apricot kernel oil.

ARAME This Japanese seaweed is a slightly larger form of hiziki (see *Hiziki*).

ARROWROOT STARCH Arrowroot starch is a fine white substance that is known variously as arrowroot starch, arrowroot flour, and arrowroot powder. The arrowroot plant is a tropical perennial herb whose food value lies in its starchy rootlike rhizomes. The starch of the arrowroot is of a very fine grain—much finer than potato starch; it is thus easily digestible and suitable for invalid and infant diets (for this purpose, make a smooth paste of the arrowroot, add warm milk or water and honey to taste). Arrowroot starch can be used to thicken gravies, soups, and fruit compotes in the same manner as cornstarch.

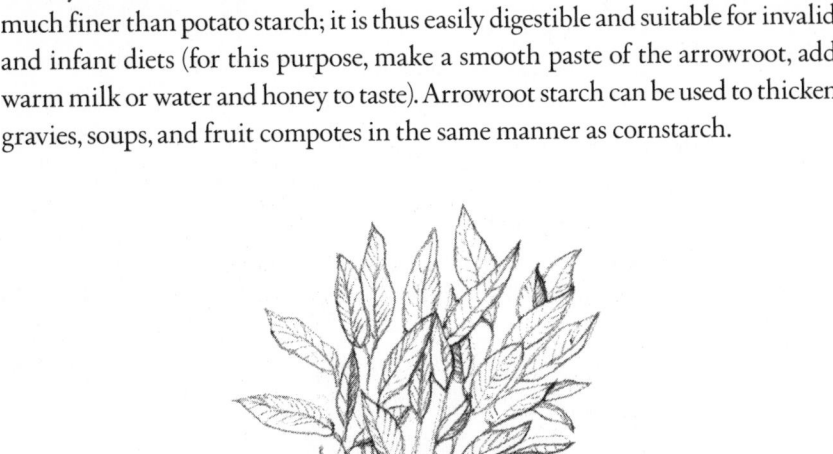

ARROWROOT
Root detail—
¼ size

ARTICHOKE NOODLE The light and tasty artichoke noodle is made from the flour of the Jerusalem artichoke, a tuber-bearing type of sunflower that was native to North America before being introduced into Europe in the seventeenth century. The unlikely name (for it is neither from Jerusalem nor in the least resembles an artichoke) seems to have derived in part from the Spanish word for "sunflower," *girasole*; as for "artichoke," its derivation is a mystery! The tuber, which looks somewhat like a small potato, is rich in iron and insulin, a sugar that can be eaten by diabetics. Jerusalem artichoke noodles also have a far lower carbohydrate content than noodles made of hard wheat.

ASTRAGALUS   Also known as *Huang Qi*, this beautiful perennial, which is native to Mongolia and China, has been utilized in Chinese medicine for thousands of years. The dried root is said to help in cases of digestive disturbances, chronic fatigue, anemia, cold, flu, high blood pressure and blood sugar levels, and in the treatment of allergies. Astragalus can be boiled as tea or taken as a tincture and is a safe, immune-system-boosting herb for children.

When purchasing any immune-boosting and post-onset cold or flu tincture, it is well worth it to make sure that astragalus is on the list of ingredients. Astragalus is known to be a vital and powerful herb for healing in its own right, as well as enhancing the healing power of the other herbs it might be paired with.

AVOCADO OIL   An ingredient in cosmetics, this pure fruit oil is also sold as a salad or cooking oil. It is most often mixed with other vegetable oils—used alone it would be like pouring liquid gold on your lettuce, for it is an expensive item. For use as a cosmetic, you will save money by buying the edible oil, instead of an expensive cosmetic preparation. Considered one of the most penetrating of all oils, it is a marvelous skin softener.

B

BAKING POWDER   Baking powder is used as a leavening agent in cookies and quick breads. Made up of an acid, a base, and a filler—for instance, baking soda, cream of tartar, and cornstarch—baking powder releases carbon dioxide bubbles that cause batter or dough to rise. Baking powder can be a dangerous product. Most commercial brands contain aluminum compounds, which should not be used for human consumption. Less objectionable, but nevertheless harmful for many people, is the high sodium content of many baking powders. So if you want to use this product, check your labels carefully. Health food stores generally carry low-sodium, aluminum-free brands of baking powder.

BAKING SODA   Best known for its use as a leavening agent in baked goods, baking soda is useful for a host of other applications that go far beyond refreshing the refrigerator and freezer. Baking soda, or sodium bicarbonate, is a naturally occurring substance derived from soda ash that regulates pH balance, thereby keeping substances from being either too acidic or too alkaline. Baking soda reacts with the acidic ingredients in batter to give off carbon dioxide, which causes the batter or dough to rise. When there are no acidic ingredients present, baking soda will not react and it is necessary to use baking powder, which contains its own acidic reactant.

Baking soda can be used to clean everything from toilet bowls to tarnished silver. Use to deodorize shoes, carpets, and closets. Clean coffee pots, scrub crayon from the walls, and brush teeth with it. A paste made from baking soda will soothe bee stings, insect bites, and poison oak.

Children can be entertained with a homemade volcano made from apple-cider vinegar and a few tablespoons of baking soda—throw in some food coloring for real excitement and watch it all erupt!

BALACHAN   Commonly used as a flavoring in Southeast Asian dishes, balachan is made from shrimp, sardines, and other small salted fish that have been fermented in the sun. Balachan is available as a paste, powder, or cake.

BALM   Balm tea, which is also known as lemon balm and Melissa tea (from its botanical name *Melissa officinalis*), has a delicate lemon-mint flavor and is valued as a carminative and a reducer of fever. Long considered to be one of the most restorative and soothing of herbs, lemon balm is worthy of cultivation in the garden patch and can be used fresh in teas. Lemon balm is said to soothe the digestion, calm the nerves, and help in the fighting of herpes simplex virus.

The leaves of sweet-smelling lemon balm are commonly used for teas, tinctures, and essential oils. A lemon balm tincture can be administered to the upset or overwrought child, or similarly to soothe the nerves of the overworked parent, and the dried leaves can be mixed with peppermint or chamomile to create a relaxing tea blend. Use 1 teaspoon of dried leaves to 2 cups of boiling water. Balm tea has value as a nerve soother, and an Arabian proverb goes even further: balm tea "makes the heart merry and joyful!" If you plan on living a hundred years, this gentle tea might help you reach your goal, for legend tells that balm wards off old age.

Fresh or dried balm will impart a delicious lemony flavor to fish, lamb, and poultry stuffing; or sprinkle it on your salad.

BANANA, DRIED   The banana is the fruit of a giant tropical herb that can grow to a height of 30 feet. After each harvest the "tree" dies and its roots send up another enormous shoot. When unripe, the banana is a very starchy food, and a nutritious, easily digested flour is made from it; this is rarely exported. As the fruit ripens, black specks appear on its surface, indicating that the starch is turning to sugar—from which point the banana is deliciously edible. The less ripe the banana, the more constipating it is; the more ripe, the more laxative it becomes.

The ripe fruit can be dried to produce a compact energy-giving food that is extremely rich in potassium and magnesium. It is also high in calories; these are not empty calories, however, but are full of nutrients. Dried banana flakes are also available, and these can be sprinkled on cereal or yogurt dishes.

BANCHA TWIG TEA   This is Japanese green tea made from tea leaves that have been aged three years on the tree—hence its brown color. Roast in a heavy skillet until an aroma arises. The tea can then be stored in a tightly sealed jar and used as needed. Add a generous pinch of roasted bancha twig tea to a quart of water (use an enamel pot or pan) and boil gently for 20 minutes; strain and serve. When a dash of soy sauce is added, this makes a very bracing, strengthening tea.

BARLEY, PEARLED   To produce pearled barley, the bran is removed from the barley grain. This is an inferior product to the whole hulled variety, and is best used in times of illness when other foods cannot be tolerated. It is the mildest and least irritating of cereal foods.

BARLEY, WHOLE HULLED   Pliny wrote in Roman times that barley was the oldest cultivated grain. Modern investigation tends to bear out his opinion; deposits of barley have been found in Stone Age lake dwellings in Switzerland. An extremely hardy grain that can withstand extremes of temperature, barley is grown as far north as the Arctic Circle and flourishes in subtropical countries as well. Barley malt has been used since prehistoric times in beer making.

Whole hulled barley is the most nutritious form of this grain, for it still bears its bran coating, which is high in B vitamins. Barley is most delicious when added to stews and soups; it lends a satisfying creamy texture. See also *Barley, Pearled.*

❦ BARLEY-BEEF SOUP

    2 pounds short ribs of beef, cut in 3-inch pieces
    2½ quarts water
    ¼ cups barley, whole hulled
    2 bay leaves
    Salt and pepper to taste
    1 cup each of any 4 chopped fresh vegetables, such as:
    onions
    carrots
    celery
    green beans
    tomatoes
    peeled and seeded zucchini, etc.
    6-8 tablespoons olive oil

  Simmer short ribs in water for 3 hours until just tender. Do this the day before serving, refrigerate the pot overnight, then skim off congealed fat and continue soup. If you prepare the beef the morning before serving, put in freezer for 1–2 hours, and fat will rise enough for thorough skimming.

Put soup back on stove. Add washed barley, bay leaves, salt, and pepper and simmer 1 hour. Meanwhile chop fresh vegetables and sauté briefly in olive oil; add and simmer 30 minutes more, until everything is tender. Taste for seasoning.

Serves six.

BARLEY FLOUR   The best barley flour is ground from whole hulled barley. When added to bread recipes, barley flour gives a moist, cakelike texture. The barley-orange bread below is useful for the allergy-prone, for it is wheat- and milk-free—and also tastes good.

BARLEY-ORANGE BREAD

2 eggs, well beaten
$\frac{1}{2}$ cup fresh-squeezed orange juice
2 tablespoons olive oil
$\frac{1}{2}$ cup honey
$\frac{1}{2}$ cup water
$\frac{1}{4}$ cup orange zest (from organic undyed oranges)
2 cups barley flour
$\frac{2}{3}$ cups sugar (preferably raw sugar)
$\frac{1}{2}$ teaspoon salt
3 teaspoons baking powder

Preheat oven to 350 degrees. Oil and flour a bread pan.

Mix together eggs, orange juice, oil, honey, water, and orange zest. Sift together flour, sugar, salt, and baking powder. Stir wet mixture into dry, beating well.

Pour into well-oiled and floured bread pan. Bake for about 70 minutes or until a knife inserted into the centers comes out clean. This is a moist sweet bread, perfect for tea or dessert.

BARLEY GRITS   Coarsely ground whole barley forms a type of grits that is quickly cooked and particularly good as a morning cereal.

BARLEY MALT SYRUP   This healthy alternative to corn syrup is processed from sprouted barley. Barley malt is made up primarily of complex sugars, which are slowly digested, and therefore there is no rapid blood sugar fluctuation, as is common with cane sugars. In other words, the highs and lows associated with other sugars are not present. Similar in taste to molasses, barely malt syrup is half as sweet as cane sugar and recipes must be adjusted accordingly. Often used to make beer, barley malt syrup works well in breads and bagels as a source of food for the yeast.

BASIL This aromatic herb is surely a god's gift to the kitchen; and divine favor shines brilliantly upon the Mediterranean's sunny shores, where basil has long grown in great profusion. The name "basil" comes from the Greek word for "king"—so greatly did the Greeks esteem this king of herbs. *Herbe royale*, the French respectfully call it. In Italy basil serves the goddess Love; a sprig of it worn by a suitor bespeaks his loving intentions. In India, too, the herb flourishes freely and is held in reverence by the Hindus, who plant it to protect both the living and the dead. Basil can also prosper in your own summer garden or flowerpot!

In fresh or dried form, basil will lend savory flavoring to tomato dishes, soups, ragouts, sauces, sausages, and salads. The pungency of basil, unlike most other herbs, increases with cooking, so handle it with care until you learn to know it well. Basil tea makes a delicious drink, hot or cold; brew it from fresh or dried leaves, a heaping teaspoon per cup, and steep for 15 minutes.

The leaves of basil are said to be antiseptic; either the fresh leaf or a decoction of the dried leaf is soothing to insect bites and stings.

TOMATOES STUFFED WITH BASIL AND RICE

4 good-sized firm tomatoes

1 cup cooked rice

2 tablespoons chopped fresh basil (or 1 tablespoon dried)

2 tablespoons chopped fresh parsley (or 1 tablespoon dried)

2 cloves garlic, finely chopped

1½ teaspoons olive oil

1 teaspoon salt

- Preheat the oven to 350 degrees.
- Cut a lid off the top of each tomato and set aside. Scoop out the inside pulp, taking care not to weaken the walls. Chop the tomato pulp and mix with the other ingredients.
- Stuff the tomatoes with the mixture, put tomato tops back on as lids, and place in an uncovered baking dish. Bake for 30 minutes. These tomatoes can be served hot, but are particularly delicious cold, and their flavor blossoms after a day or so of refrigeration.
- Serves four.

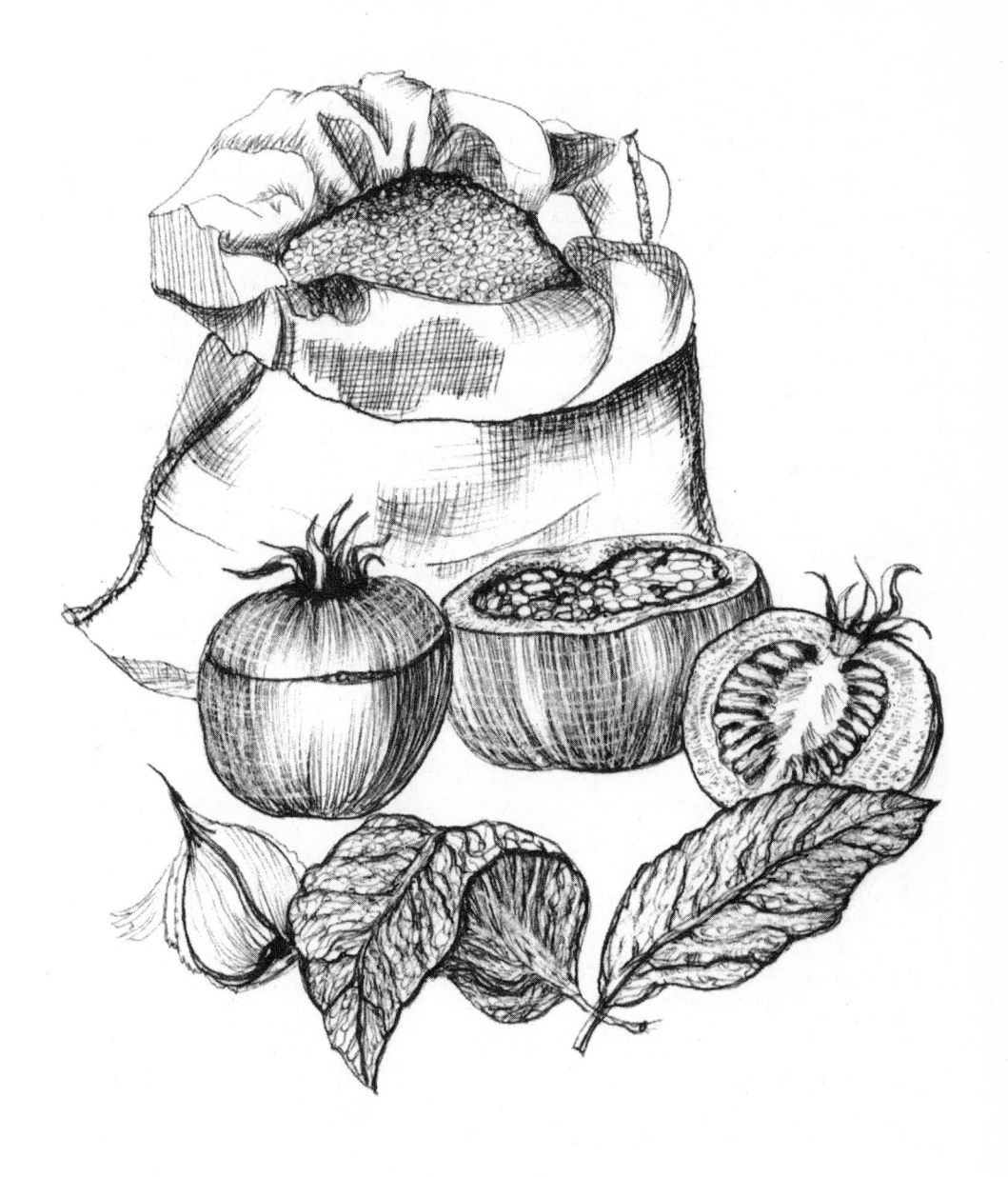

PESTO ALLA GENOVESE

    36 leaves fresh basil (or 2 tablespoons dried)
    1 garlic clove
    1 handful pignoli nuts (or walnuts)
    2 tablespoons grated Parmesan cheese
    ½ teaspoon salt
    ½ teaspoon freshly ground black pepper
    ⅔ cup olive oil

- Finely chop basil, garlic, and nuts (or pulverize in mortar). Put in a small bowl, stir in Parmesan, salt and pepper, then oil. (Or put all ingredients into a blender, but the sauce will lose some texture.)
- This pesto is a superb sauce for spaghetti (enough for 1 pound). It can also be added to vegetable or bean soups with most appetizing results.

TOMATO BASIL SOUP

    3 tablespoons olive oil
    5 cloves garlic, chopped
    3 pounds fresh tomatoes, peeled, seeded, and finely chopped, or
        3 large cans peeled plum tomatoes, seeded, and finely
        chopped
    1 cup fresh basil leaves, shredded
    5 cups chicken or vegetable stock
    Salt and pepper

- Heat olive oil over medium heat in a medium saucepan. Sauté garlic. Add tomatoes. Cook for 5 minutes. Add basil, chicken stock, salt, and pepper. Bring to a boil. Reduce to a simmer. Cook for 30–40 minutes. Purée this mixture with a hand wand, Cuisinart, or blender. You may choose not to purée it at all, if you prefer. Serve cold or hot.
- Serves four to six.

BAY LEAF   The bay laurel tree is actually a large evergreen shrub. Its history is a lengthy and noble one; among the ancient Greek the laurel tree was sacred to the god Apollo. A wreath of its branches became the symbol of victory—in war, athletic games, and literary contests—and today we still have our poet laureates. Legend has it that lightning will never strike a bay laurel tree, and the emperor Tiberius is said to have worn a laurel wreath on his head during thunderstorms. Well—it wouldn't hurt to try!

Bay leaves are very pungent in the cooking pot, so be stingy with them. One leaf will lend its characteristic bitter taste to a stew or soup for four people. Remove the leaf before serving, because no amount of cooking will render it tender enough to eat.

Use a bay leaf in your marinade, or when preparing fish stock. And of course the crumbled bay leaf is essential to a bouquet garni, bagged or tied herbs that are added to soups, stews, and broths for added flavor and then later removed.

BEANS, DRIED   Dried beans are available to us in a most fantastic variety—fava beans, pinto beans, kidney beans, mung beans, soybeans, marrow beans, split yellow peas, split green peas, whole peas, cowpeas, chickpeas, adzuki beans … the list could go on and on. Beans offer an extremely good source of protein, niacin, vitamins B_1 and B_2, as well as valuable minerals such as iron, magnesium, sodium, and calcium. Their protein content makes them an excellent meat substitute. With a dozen glass jars of different beans (for why not display their beauty rather than tuck them away in a dark cupboard) in your kitchen, you will be able to give any one basic recipe twelve completely different faces. And dried beans are inexpensive! Those that are organically grown cost more than those that are chemically grown, of course, but their superior flavor usually makes the additional cost worthwhile.

Tips on cooking dried beans: With the exception of split peas and lentils, all beans should be soaked overnight before cooking. Or instead of long soaking, bring beans and water to a rolling boil, then turn off heat and soak for 2 hours; use as needed. One cupful of dried beans will swell in bulk to feed about four people. Cook beans slowly so that they do not burst and lose their shape. Slow cooking also cuts down on the gas-producing tendencies of dried beans. See also individual beans.

🌿 BEAN SOUP

1 cup white beans, dried (or kidney beans, fava beans, pinto beans, chickpeas, etc.)

3 quarts water (or vegetable or meat broth)

Ham bone, or ½ pound diced salt pork or prosciutto ends (optional)

1 bay leaf

3 tablespoons olive oil

8 cups any assorted fresh vegetables on hand:

chopped onions

sliced carrots

sliced zucchini

diced eggplant

diced string beans

diced tomatoes

peas, etc.

1 cup macaroni

Salt and pepper to taste

2 tablespoons chopped parsley

- Soak beans in 1 quart water overnight. Do not throw out the soaking water. In a large saucepan combine soaked beans, another 2 quarts water or broth, bone or meat if you use it, and bay leaf, and simmer slowly until beans are almost tender (about 3 hours).

- Sauté freshly chopped vegetables in oil and add to soup. Add macaroni, salt, and pepper, and simmer 30 minutes until everything is tender. Add parsley and serve. Or let the soup stand for a few hours before serving; its taste will be even fuller.

- Serves four to six.

BEE POLLEN   Produced by bees to feed their young, bee pollen is rich in minerals, amino acids, enzymes, and vitamins B complex, A, C, D, E, and beta-carotene. Bee pollen is collected from male seed flowers, mixed with secretions from the bee, and formed into golden granules that melt in the mouth. Bee pollen is said to be useful in relieving respiratory problems and is believed by many to be an essential additive to the diet during allergy season. Keep in mind, however, that to alleviate allergies, *local* bee pollen must be purchased. Otherwise the bee pollen will not necessarily have been harvested from the plants in your area that are causing such grief to the sinuses, so while the nutritional benefits will still be present, the level of relief may not be the same.

Bee pollen should be stored in the refrigerator, or even better, the freezer, and can be mixed with smoothies or eaten straight from the jar. A dosage of 1–2 teaspoons a day is recommended, and don't feel surprised if you feel a burst of energy after its consumption. Bee pollen is reputed to counteract the effects of aging and increase both mental and physical strength.

BEE PROPOLIS   Yet another astounding by-product of the honeybee, propolis is collected by bees from the resin underneath tree bark. The strong antibiotic, antiviral, and antifungal properties of propolis make it indispensable when treating a variety of health concerns, both internal and external. Propolis is said to be beneficial in the treatment of stomach ulcers, warts, herpes lesions, toothaches, gum healing, and for boosting the immune system. High in bioflavonoids, amino acids, trace minerals—such as calcium, magnesium, and zinc—B-vitamins, and vitamins E, C, and beta-carotene.

Propolis is available in a thick, concentrated tincture that can be used topically on warts, herpes, and other sores, as well as applied directly to an infected tooth. But be prepared—this form of propolis is tarlike—very dark and sticky. A more soluble concentration is available for mixing with liquid and taken internally, and lozenges can be chewed for the benefit of mouth, gums, and throat.

BLACK COHOSH   Also known as rattlesnake or squawroot, this perennial herb (*Cimicifuga racemosa*) is native to the United States. Hearsay has it that the root contains an antidote for rattlesnake poison. Proven to be extremely effective in relieving menopausal symptoms, black cohosh is also useful in cases of arthritis, cramps, and back pain. Black cohosh is available as a tea, tincture, and capsule. Avoid during pregnancy, as black cohosh can bring on uterine contractions. Do not use this herb while nursing.

To brew the tea, steep 1 teaspoonful of the chopped dried root in 1 cup boiling water for 15 minutes.

BLACKSTRAP MOLASSES   See *Molasses*.

BLADDER WRACK   Bladder wrack is a common seaweed that grows attached to rocks rather than to the sea bottom. It is rich in iodine and trace minerals. Bladder wrack, which is often referred to as kelp, is said to be helpful in the treatment of thyroid problems as well as for weight loss and balancing the metabolism. Bladder wrack is available as a tea, tincture, or capsule. As there is a risk of heavy metal contamination, be sure to purchase bladder wrack that is certified heavy metal–free.

Although harvesting one's own seaweeds may seem tempting, just as when mushroom hunting, certain practices must be followed in order to ensure personal safety. Therefore, it is best to study up before attempting to harvest seaweeds from the wild.

BLUE COHOSH   Also known as the papoose root, blue cohosh was traditionally valued by Native Americans for its incredible ability to stimulate uterine contractions. Useful during the last few weeks of pregnancy only, blue cohosh is said to speed labor as well as relieve both labor pains and menstrual cramps. The roots and rhizome are available as a tincture, tea, or capsule, but avoid the berries, as they are poisonous!

BLUEBERRY JUICE   Wild bears will eat nothing but blueberries when they are in season, sometimes traveling ten to fifteen miles per day on an empty stomach just to sniff out a blueberry patch. The bears must be onto something, because blueberries are becoming increasingly well known for their health benefits. Unfortunately, blueberry juice does not come cheap, and will probably never become available in the gallon juice jugs that apple juice so commonly frequents. Too bad for us, because blueberry juice is both delicious and healthful!

Like cranberry juice, blueberry juice is reputed to be useful in combating urinary tract infections, as it keeps bacteria form adhering to the bladder wall. Packed with antioxidants, blueberry juice is also said to dramatically improve night vision and to protect against cataracts and glaucoma. Half a cup of blueberry juice delivers as much antioxidant power as five servings of fruits and vegetables and is said to protect against both aging and cancer. Not the blueberry season? Try squeezing extra blueberries into the diet by using organic frozen blueberries in smoothies!

🌿 FRUIT TART

        1 pint blueberries or 6–8 peaches (or a mixture of both!)
        ½ cup plus 2 tablespoons sugar (preferably raw sugar)
        1 cup plus 2 tablespoons unbleached white flour
        ½ teaspoon cinnamon
        Butter, 8 tablespoons (1 stick), softened, cut into pieces
        1 tablespoon white vinegar

- Preheat oven to 400 degrees. Butter a 9-inch fluted tart pan with a drop-out bottom.
- Mix chosen fruit with ½ cup sugar, 2 tablespoons flour, and cinnamon. Set aside.
- Spin in a food processor for 30 seconds: 1 cup flour, 2 tablespoons sugar, and the butter. Slowly add 1 tablespoon vinegar while spinning, until dough makes a ball. Press into the prepared pan. Arrange fruit on top and bake for 45 minutes.
- Serve warm as is or topped with fresh-made whipping cream. The tart can also be served chilled.
- Serves six to eight.

BLUEBERRY TEA   This tea is made from the dried, crushed leaves of the blueberry bush. When taken regularly and over a long period of time, it is said to be an effective remedy for diabetes as well as for healing urinary tract infections. Steep 1 teaspoon dried leaves in 2 cups boiling water for 20 minutes.

BORAGE   A beautiful addition to any garden, borage has tall furry stalks topped with small, purple, star-shaped flowers that can be added to salads or used as an edible decoration for cakes and deserts. Be aware, however, that once introduced to the garden, borage can spread quite rampantly and provides an irresistible draw for honeybees. The leaves of the borage plant can be used in salads or cooked like any other leafy green. The stalks can be peeled and used as one would a cucumber.

High in gamma-linolenic acid, or GLA, an essential fatty acid, borage seed oil is a healthy addition to the diet and can often be found in conjunction with flax and primrose oils. Borage seed oil is said to ease menstrual problems, skin breakouts, and irritable bowel syndrome. Borage is regarded as an uplifting plant, good for the mood and emotions, and can be taken as a tincture or, should fresh leaves be available, as a tea. The leaves can also be used as a poultice to soothe a variety of skin irritations.

BRAN   Bran is the outer coating of the wheat kernel; in it are concentrated valuable amounts of minerals and vitamin B. In making commercial flours and breads, the bran is almost always removed.

There are problems with bran, however. Pesticides are said to be strongly concentrated in the bran layer of the wheat kernel. Therefore, take care that your whole wheat flour is organically grown. Certain people with peptic ulcers or intestinal problems find bran difficult to tolerate. There is a way around this: when making your whole wheat bread, mix everything except the yeast, keeping the mixture rather moist, and let it stand overnight; in the morning add the yeast dissolved in a little water, and knead well, using unbleached white flour for dusting. You will find that this method also overcomes problems of dryness and crumbling in the bread.

Bran is sometimes recommended as a laxative. Be careful, however, for bran can be an intestinal irritant unless properly soaked or cooked.

BRAZIL NUT   The Brazil nut is the fruit of a tall South American tree. Each of its large woody fruits carries a dozen to two dozen nuts inside, arranged like the sections of an orange. The individual nuts also have a very hard covering—as anyone who has struggled to crack one can vouch. Brazil nuts are high in phosphorus, protein, and unsaturated oils. They are a concentrated nutrient and should be eaten sparingly and chewed well. Delicious nut butter can be made by grinding the Brazil nut either alone or with cashew nuts; like all pure nut butters, this should be kept refrigerated.

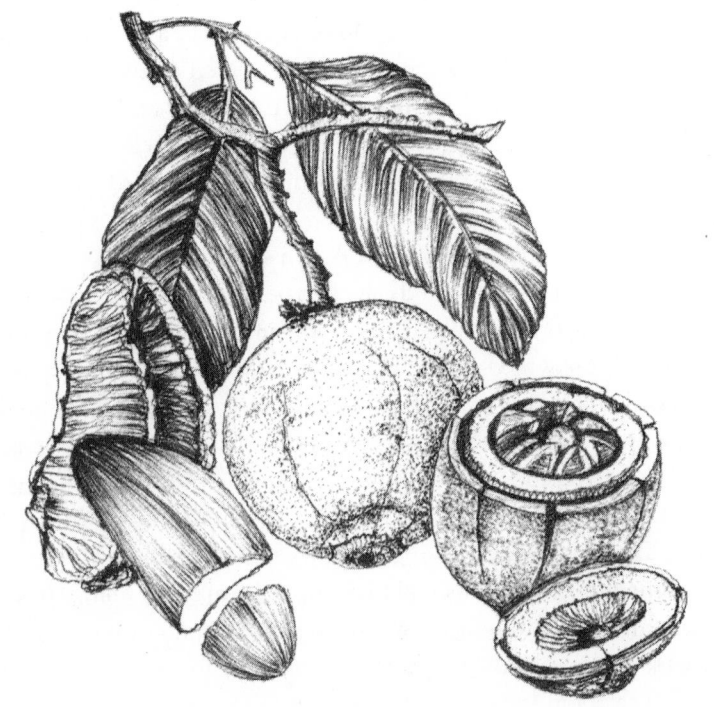

BRAZIL NUT
Nut and Kernel—
life size
Fruit, complete and in
sections—½ size

BREAD   In Roman times, whiteness of bread carried an "upper class" connotation; dark bread was the fare of the common people. For in those days it was far easier simply to use whole ground wheat kernel for bread than to sift and bolt and age the flour to attain a whiter color. Today, however, the tables have turned! It is now far easier and cheaper to produce lily-white bread than whole grain bread. The white bread of the rich has become the food of the people, and the dark loaf of the poor graces the tables of the well-to-do.

Expect bread made from stone-ground, organically grown wheat to be expensive. The fact that the flour is stone ground, grown without pesticides, contains the germ and bran of the kernel, and has not been bleached adds to the expense. And all these essentials that make whole bread healthful and delectable are anathema to the industrialized food field.

Consider by contrast the manner in which bread flour is treated by the food moguls. First the grain is grown on chemically fertilized and pesticide-laden soils; next it is robbed of bran and germ, taking away its very essence and leaving primarily starch; then it is pulverized in grinding machines that reach such degrees of heat that the resulting flour is actually "precooked" (with a corresponding loss of nutrients). Finally the flour, if it can now be called so, is bleached with chlorine dioxide (a poison). This wondrous white powder is now prepared to sit for any number of years on the grocer's shelf—no fear that it will spoil or bugs will touch it—or it is made into loaves of spongy tastelessness, shot with emulsifiers to imitate eggs and cream, with dye to imitate whole wheat, with mold inhibitors, hydrogenated fats, and synthetic vitamins.

By giving up white "commercial" bread, you need not be doomed forever to the leaden loaves (nonetheless delightful to the appreciative taste) of the intrepid macrobiotic. Not at all! If your nearest natural bakery or health food store cannot satisfy your desire for a buoyant loaf that will not overpower the food that accompanies it, become a baker yourself. It is a joyous activity, and if your experimentations don't at first reach your ideal, at least they'll make the most delicious rejects going. By juggling the amounts of whole wheat flour, whole wheat pastry flour, unbleached white flour, etc., you will be able to achieve loaves as heavy or as light, as strong-flavored or as subtle-tasting, as you desire.

Bread crumbs (toss a few slices of bread in the blender and voilà!) and bread dishes take on an extra dimension when made with whole grain bread. Try the easy "soufflé" below and you will see.

GOLDEN CHEESE "SOUFFLÉ"

2 eggs

2 cups milk (part of this can be cream if extra richness is desired)

½ teaspoon salt

½ teaspoon paprika

½ teaspoon dry mustard

3 teaspoons minced onion

2 tablespoons butter, melted

6 slices whole grain bread (or more, if needed)

¼ pound cheddar cheese, grated

¼ pound Parmesan cheese, grated

- Preheat oven to 325 degrees.
- Beat together eggs, milk, salt, paprika, mustard, and onion. Put melted butter in bottom of a shallow baking dish. Arrange alternating layers of sliced bread, mixed grated cheeses, and egg mixture, ending with grated cheese on top. Bake 45 minutes at 325 degrees.
- Serves four.

BREWER'S YEAST   This yeast, also known as nutritional yeast, was originally a by-product of the brewing industry—hence its name. Today, however, it is grown specifically for human consumption and is a rich source of vitamin B, containing all the elements of the B complex and a large amount of protein. Great for instant pep and sustained energy, it is a boon to those who watch their weight, for it contains little fat, carbohydrates, or sugar—it will not make you lose weight, but it will give you the energy to zip off unwanted poundage. If you are deficient in the B vitamins, you may find that brewer's yeast at first produces gas; therefore, work up to a good dosage gradually, starting with a teaspoonful or less. Shop around for a brand of yeast that is palatable to you; if you can't stomach one kind, give it to your pets (in small amounts, it helps to control fleas), and try again!

Brewer's yeast comes in powder, flake, and pill form. The flakes dissolve more easily than the powder, and the pills are convenient for travelers, but the powder is far more concentrated than either and offers an immediate pickup that is too good to be missed.

Brewer's yeast can also be added in small amounts to breads, soups, stews, meat loaves, etc. A caution: Do not confuse this yeast, whose growth has been arrested by heating, with baking yeast, which is a live substance that may continue growing in the intestines with deleterious results.

❦ PAN-FRIED TOFU WITH NUTRITIONAL YEAST
1 pound firm tofu
2 eggs
1 cup nutritional yeast
2–4 tablespoons olive oil
Soy sauce

• Dice tofu into small ½-inch squares. Beat eggs in bowl and lay out nutritional yeast on a large plate. Alternately dip tofu pieces in egg and then roll in nutritional yeast until coated.

• Heat desired amount of olive oil in skillet over medium-high heat and toss in the egg-and-yeast-coated tofu. Allow tofu to fry, turning occasionally with a spatula until tofu becomes golden brown. After 8 minutes of cooking, begin to sprinkle with soy sauce and then turn with a spatula. Sprinkle with soy sauce and turn until the tofu is crispy and golden.

• Serve immediately with vegetable stir-fry or over rice.

• Serves four.

❦ NUTRITIONAL YEAST POPCORN
1 cup popcorn, popped
4 tablespoons (½ stick) unsalted butter, melted
½ cup nutritional yeast
Soy sauce to taste

• Toss popcorn with melted butter and nutritional yeast, and sprinkle with a bit of soy sauce. Go easy on the soy sauce, as both the soy and the nutritional yeast are quite salty. This is a great way to get the kids to eat nutritional yeast, as they almost always love this combination.

BUCKWHEAT   A hardy grasslike herb, buckwheat produces a three-cornered seed, known as kasha or buckwheat groats, that is used in much the same manner as grain. High in potassium and phosphorus, buckwheat contains all eight essential amino acids and is particularly high in lysine. Buckwheat is a staple in Russia and in Brittany, but it is not so commonly used in the United States. That is unfortunate, for buckwheat is one of the few commercially grown products that are not routinely doused with insecticides—for its extreme hardiness makes it almost blight-free. Buckwheat is grown extensively for honey making; dark and flavorful, it yields one of the most nutritious of honeys.

Buckwheat groats are generally available roasted or raw. If you enjoy a really fresh-roasted flavor, buy the raw groats and roast them yourself; just put them in a heavy frying pan over medium heat and stir until browned on all sides. Kasha (as roasted buckwheat groats are more usually called) can be served as a warming breakfast cereal, with honey and cream added. It can also be used as stuffing for game or fowl, or served as a rice substitute. If you find the pungent musty flavor of kasha a little strange at first, try mixing it with rice.

KASHA WITH RICE

4 cups water
1½ teaspoons salt
1 cup brown rice
1 egg
1 cup kasha (roasted)
1 tablespoon butter

- Bring salted water to boil. Meanwhile wash brown rice in a sieve and drain it. When water reaches rolling boil, sprinkle rice in slowly enough so that the water does not stop boiling. Cover tightly.
- Beat egg and mix with kasha until all grains are coated. In a hot heavy frying pan stir this mixture briskly until each grain of kasha is dry and separate. When rice has been cooking for 15 minutes, add the kasha to it and cover. Cook for 30 minutes more, until liquid is absorbed and kasha and rice are tender. Add butter.
- Serve as a side dish with fresh steamed vegetables or fish.
- Serves four.

BUCKWHEAT FLOUR   This gray flour speckled with black is traditionally used in the United States for making buckwheat pancakes. Their Russian counterpart—blini—is not limited to the breakfast table; served with red caviar and sour cream, they render any meal exotic. Buckwheat flour can also be added to bread recipes in small amounts (approximately ½ cup buckwheat flour to 4 cups wheat flour). Because it contains no gluten, buckwheat flour will not rise on its own. Buckwheat flour will produce a dense but deliciously moist bread. See also *Buckwheat*.

BLINI (BUCKWHEAT PANCAKES)

1 cup milk

1/2 cup water

2 tablespoons pressed vegetable oil or melted butter

2 tablespoons honey

1 egg

1/2 cup buckwheat flour

1/2 cup whole wheat pastry flour

2 teaspoons baking powder

1/2 teaspoon salt

- Beat together milk, water, oil, honey, and egg. Sift dry ingredients into liquid mixture and stir just enough to dampen the flour; do not overbeat. The batter should be rather thin.

- To cook, lightly oil a cast-iron griddle or heavy frying pan. Heat over medium heat until drops of water sprinkled on it dance. Spoon batter onto griddle; cook until bubbly on top, then turn over and brown the other side. Try not to turn more than once.

- Serve hot with butter and maple syrup; or with butter, sour cream, and red caviar; or with sugared ricotta.

- Makes 21 six-inch blini.

BUCKWHEAT GRITS   Coarsely ground buckwheat grits make an ideal winter cereal and are quicker cooking than the whole groats. See also *Buckwheat*.

BUCKWHEAT GROATS   See *Buckwheat*.

BULGUR   Bulgur is to the Middle East what rice is to Asia and kasha is to Russia. It is a cracked wheat that retains the bran and germ of the grain. In olden times it was roasted in open braziers, dried in the sun, then cracked in a mortar and pestle. Today the methods have been mechanized, but the basic process remains the same.

Bulgur is a most versatile grain and very simple to prepare. Everything from salads to cereals takes on new interest when bulgur is used.

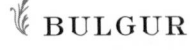 BULGUR

    1 medium-size onion, sliced thin
    2 tablespoons olive oil
    1 cup bulgur
    2 cups chicken or vegetable broth (or water)
    1 teaspoon salt

- Gently sauté onion in oil in a medium saucepan for about 3 minutes. Add bulgur and stir to coat all grains with oil. Add broth and salt, and bring to a boil. Cover and turn heat down to simmering. Cook about 20 minutes or until liquid is absorbed and bulgur is fluffy.
- Serve as a substitute for rice or potatoes.
- Serves four.

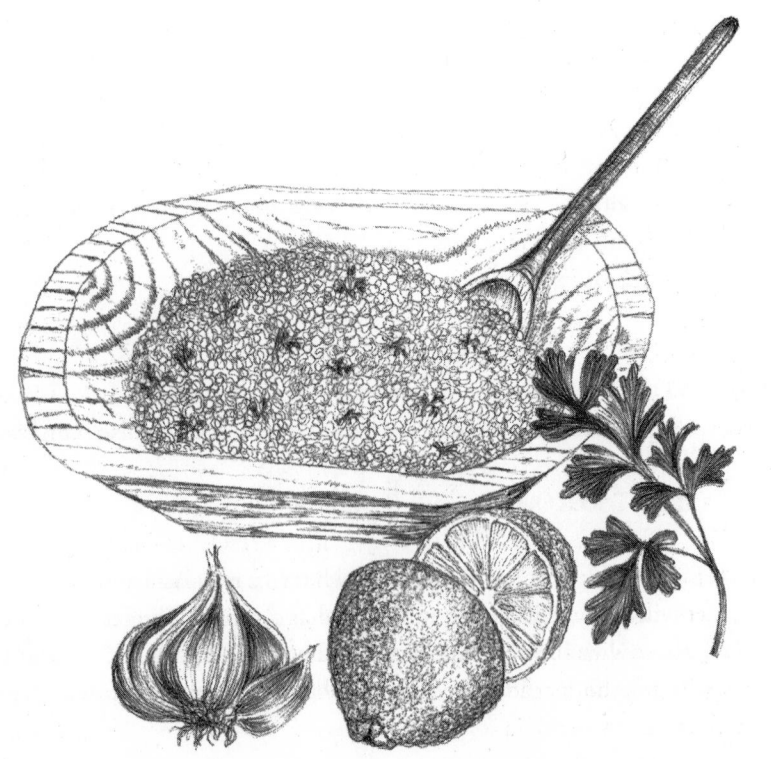

TABBOULEH (BULGUR AND PARSLEY SALAD)

$^3/_4$ cup bulgur

1 cup boiling water

1 clove garlic, finely chopped

$^1/_2$ cup fresh mint, finely chopped (or 2 tablespoons dried)

$1^1/_2$ cups fresh Italian parsley, chopped (or $^1/_2$ cup dried)

3 chopped tomatoes

1 teaspoon salt

$^1/_2$ teaspoon pepper

$^1/_2$ cup lemon juice

$^1/_2$ cup olive oil

Soak bulgur in 1 cup boiling water for 30 minutes or until water is absorbed. Mix in chopped ingredients, then add salt and pepper, lemon juice, and olive oil.

Serves four.

BURDOCK   In Japan and Hawaii, the importance of burdock root (also known as *gobo*) is well appreciated and the plant is extensively cultivated. In the United States, burdock (*Arctium lappa*) is regarded as an all-too-common and pesky weed. If you do not come across this large-leafed plant in your backyard, try an Asian market or a health food store. There you will be sure to find the long, skinny burdock root, which is a common ingredient of *nituke*—sautéed vegetables, Japanese style. The tender young stems of burdock may also be eaten— peeled and steamed and served with butter, yielding a delicious vegetable much like asparagus.

Tea prepared from either the root or the seed of the burdock is said to be an extremely effective blood purifier. As such, it is reputedly helpful in remedying skin disorders and rheumatic pains. Steep 1 teaspoon dried root in 1 cup boiling water for 5 minutes. Strain and serve with honey if desired.

BURNET   The cucumber-like flavor of this native European perennial herb will enhance any salad; in fact, it is often known as salad burnet. Easy to grow, burnet will provide leaves all year round and actually prefers dry, poor soil, so even those with brown thumbs can give burnet a try! It will also add a spark to iced drinks and creamed vegetable dishes. The tea made from its dried leaves is useful as a cleansing tonic; it also has certain antiseptic qualities, is soothing when applied to skin wounds, calms the stomach, and is said to stem the flow of blood. To brew burnet tea, steep 1 teaspoon dried leaves in 2 cups boiling water for about 15 minutes.

BUTTER   While the price of organic butter may be so intimidating many will overlook it in favor of cheaper counterparts, let it be known that butter has the highest pesticide concentrations of any dairy food. Organic butter tastes better, too! Though many health proponents point their fingers at butter because of its high cholesterol and saturated fat levels, to many of us, butter is too utterly delicious to be given up. Fresh organic butter adds flavor and richness to baked goods, desserts, or a simple piece of toast that simply cannot be replicated by any butter substitute. If the price of organic butter is too much, or the taste of real, authentic fresh butter is desired, butter can be made quite easily at home using organic cream.

BUTTER IN THE BLENDER
> ½ pint heavy cream
> ½ cup ice water

- Whip cream in blender at high speed. When whipped, add ice water and continue at high speed until butter is formed (this can take a minute or two). Pour butter into sieve to drain. Do not throw away the drippings; use them in cooking. Butter can also be made in the same manner in an electric mixer.
- Makes about ½ cup butter.

PLUM TORTE
> 1 cup sugar
> 8 tablespoons (1 stick) sweet butter, softened
> 1 cup unbleached flour, sifted
> 1 teaspoon baking powder
> Pinch of salt
> 2 eggs
> 24 pitted purple plums, halved

TOPPING:
> Sugar
> Lemon juice
> Cinnamon

- ❧ Preheat oven to 350 degrees. Butter a 9-inch springform pan.
- ❧ Cream sugar and butter. Add flour, baking powder, salt, and eggs. Beat well. Spoon batter into prepared pan. Place plum halves skin side up on top of batter. Sprinkle lightly with sugar and lemon juice, depending upon sweetness of fruit. Sprinkle with about 1 teaspoon of cinnamon, to taste.
- ❧ Bake at 350 degrees for 1 hour. Remove and cool. Refrigerate or freeze if desired, or cool to lukewarm.
- ❧ Serve plain or with vanilla ice cream or whipped cream. To serve frozen torte, defrost and reheat briefly at 300 degrees.
- ❧ Serves eight.

FALL APPLE CAKE

　　2 cups unbleached white flour
　　½ teaspoon salt
　　1 teaspoon ground allspice
　　1 teaspoon ground cinnamon
　　1 teaspoon ground nutmeg
　　¼ teaspoon ground cloves
　　1¼ cups sugar
　　8 tablespoons (1 stick) butter, softened
　　2 eggs
　　1 cup cold strong coffee
　　1 teaspoon baking soda
　　2½–3 cups tart and firm apples, peeled and sliced
　　1 cup raisins
　　1 cup walnuts, chopped

FROSTING:

　　1 cup powdered sugar
　　3 spoonfuls of the strong coffee made for the cake

- ❧ Preheat oven to 350 degrees. Grease and line a 9 x 9 x 2-inch pan with parchment. Sift flour, salt, and spices. Set aside. In a separate large bowl cream butter and sugar together. Add eggs to the creamed mixture and beat well. Dissolve the baking soda in the coffee. Slowly add the flour to the butter and eggs with the coffee. Fold in the apples, raisins, and nuts. Bake for 40–45 minutes or until knife inserted in middle comes out clean.

🍂 To make frosting, mix powdered sugar with coffee to desired consistency. Spread on cake. You may garnish it with a few extra nuts on top if you wish.

BUTTERMILK   In foregone times, buttermilk was the natural by-product of butter making. As cream was churned, butter separated from it, leaving a thick, low-fat acidulous milk flecked with bits of butter. This was drained off by removing a plug from the bottom of the churn. Today's buttermilk usually has nothing to do with butter. It is an imitation of what it used to be, and is made from skim milk with culture added to give acidity, and flecks of butter thrown in for nostalgia's sake. It is a healthful product, low in fat, high in calcium—but it is not buttermilk! Certified raw buttermilk is to be preferred over the pasteurized kind—if you can find it.

Buttermilk is often recommended for pregnant and nursing women. Although it is low in fat, it provides the acid and enough fat to increase absorption of much-needed calcium and is high in B vitamins.

🌿 BUTTERMILK WAFFLES

1 cup stone-ground whole wheat flour
1 cup unbleached white flour
$\frac{1}{3}$ cup toasted wheat germ
$\frac{1}{2}$ teaspoon salt
2 teaspoons baking powder
$1\frac{1}{2}$ teaspoons baking soda
4 tablespoons ($\frac{1}{2}$ stick) butter
3 large eggs
2 cups buttermilk

🍂 Mix all dry ingredients together. Melt butter and cool. Beat the eggs and add to buttermilk. Mix together with cooled butter. Add wet mixture to the dry and mix together. Do not overmix. Ladle appropriate amount of batter onto heated waffle iron. Cook until firm and somewhat crisp.

🍂 Serves four to six.

🌿 ORANGE MINI-MUFFINS

$\frac{3}{4}$ cup sugar
8 tablespoons (1 stick) unsalted butter, softened

2 eggs

1 teaspoon baking soda

1 cup buttermilk

2 cups sifted all-purpose flour

½ teaspoon salt

Zest and juice of one orange (use an organic orange to avoid the
potential for dye)

½ cup sugar (optional, for topping)

🐦 Preheat oven to 400 degrees. Butter miniature muffin tins. With electric mixer, cream the sugar and butter until smooth. Add eggs and beat until fluffy. Add baking soda to the buttermilk.

🐦 Sift flour and salt, then add to the sugar-butter mix alternately with the buttermilk. Stir well. Add zest. Spoon into the tins. Bake until golden brown and firm to touch, about 12 minutes. Remove to cooling racks.

🐦 Place tins close together. Brush tops with orange juice and sprinkle with sugar while still warm. After 5 minutes, turn muffins out of pans. If you don't want them to be sweet, you can eliminate the sugar topping.

🐦 Makes at least 2 dozen mini-muffins.

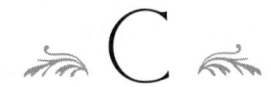

C

CANE SYRUP   Cane syrup, a by-product of sugar refining, is a thick, dark golden syrup containing more sugar than molasses. It is used primarily in the southern United States in the same manner as maple syrup is used in the north. "Organically" refined cane syrup has not been treated with the usual lime or sulfur.

CARAWAY SEED   A member of the carrot family, caraway was once used in love potions and to protect valued possessions from thieves. Native to Europe, Siberia, and the Himalayas, it is said that the farther north caraway grows, the more aromatic are the seeds. As a medicinal, 1 teaspoon bruised seeds to 2 cups boiling water gives a tea that is valued to aid in digestion and expel gas, to encourage menstruation, and to soothe the pain of a colicky infant. In cooking it is used to flavor bread, cakes and cookies, sauerkraut, and mild cheeses. Next time you serve bread and any Muenster-type cheese, put a small bowl of caraway seeds on the table; sprinkled on a slice of cheese they add delicious pungency and aroma. Caraway is also the flavor base of Kümmel liqueur.

CARDAMOM SEED   Cardamom pods, the fruit of an herbaceous plant native to India and Ceylon, contain aromatic seeds that are used to flavor desserts, mulled wines, and curries. They must be harvested carefully lest the pod split open and the seeds lose some of their heady essence. In Asia cardamom seeds are chewed to sweeten the breath; early American colonists used them for the same purpose.

CAROB POD   The flat leathery seedpods of the carob tree are sometimes called St. John's bread in reference to a belief that these pods were the "locust"

St. John fed on in the wilderness, for the honey locust tree is somewhat similar to the carob tree. The carob tree is native to the Mediterranean region; before chocolate became a common commodity, the dry carob pod was a "candy" to the poorer children of that area. Chewing carob pods may not appeal to more refined tastes, but they do yield a sugary, vaguely chocolate-like flavor and lots of nutrients in the form of minerals and vitamin A.

Carob is used nowadays mainly as a chocolate substitute for those who are allergic to chocolate or wish to avoid it because of its high fat content (carob has 2 percent fat as opposed to the 52 percent in chocolate). Carob can yield some delicious confections, but don't expect them to taste just like chocolate or you are doomed to disappointment.

CAROB POWDER   The flourlike powder of the ground carob is found toasted and raw. The toasted powder is dark brown, similar in appearance to cocoa, and this is mostly used as a chocolate substitute. As a general rule, 3 teaspoons carob powder plus 2 tablespoons liquid (water or milk) equals 1 square of unsweetened chocolate.

CARRAGEEN   See *Irish Moss.*

CASHEW NUT   The cashew nut is actually the seed of the cashew fruit, a fleshy pear-shaped "apple." The seed grows in a curious manner—it hangs, kidney-shaped, from the outside end of the fruit. The tropical cashew tree, or shrub, is native to Brazil, the West Indies, and India, as well as parts of Central and South America. The cashew "apple" is used locally as a fruit and to make a fermented liquor called *kajú*, and is reputed to be absolutely delicious, though it spoils too quickly to ever be exported. The tree is related to the poison sumac, and the shells of the nuts contain an oil that is extremely irritating to the skin—this liquid is used to make varnishes and insecticides. The hull of the cashew nut and the poison juices are removed, leaving the pale, soft, delectable nut that graces our tables.

High in unsaturated fats and protein, the cashew nut also supplies good amounts of magnesium, sodium, and iron. It is an extremely versatile nut. Because of its softness, it can easily be blended to a smooth paste and used in cream soups, milk, ice cream, and nut butter. And, of course, cashew nuts are unbeatable au naturel.

CASHEW NUT

Kernel—life size
Branch with
Fruits—⅔ size

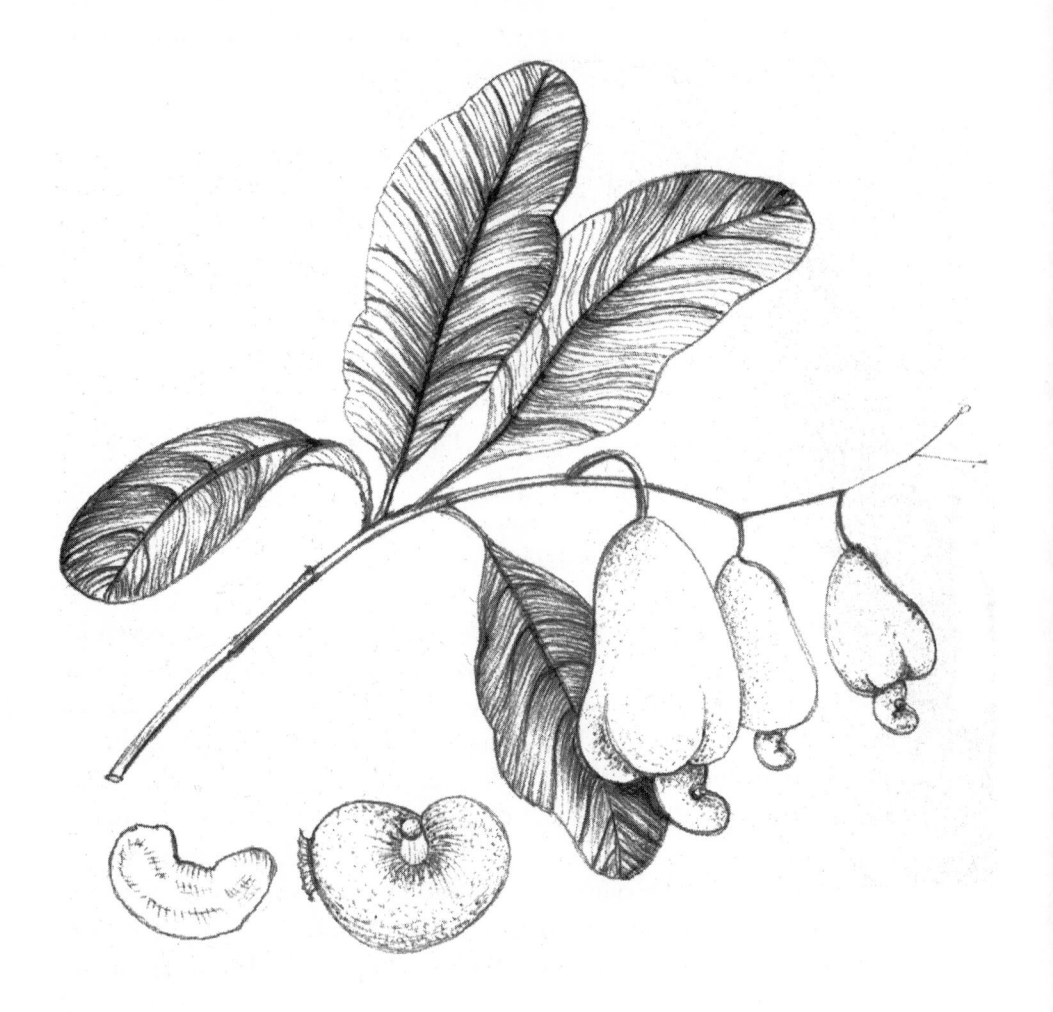

THE DICTIONARY OF WHOLESOME FOODS

CHICKEN CURRY

1 chicken, cut into 8 pieces (3½–4 pounds)
6 tablespoons olive oil
1 large onion, chopped
2 cloves garlic, chopped
1½ teaspoons coriander
½ teaspoon turmeric
2–3 teaspoons cumin
¼ teaspoon cloves
1 teaspoon ginger
¼ teaspoon cayenne (or to taste)
⅓ teaspoon cardamom
¾ cup coconut milk, unsweetened
1 teaspoon salt
3 cups plain yogurt
½ cup water
1 cup raw cashews
1 tablespoon butter
Juice of 2 limes

Brown chicken in olive oil. Remove from pan. Sautè onions and garlic, then add spices and cook for five minutes, stirring frequently. Add chicken, coconut milk, yogurt, and water. Simmer for 40 minutes (do not boil, or yogurt will curdle). While simmering, sauté cashews in butter. Add cashews and lime juice to chicken. Serve on basmati rice.

Serves four.

CATNIP   Cats should not be given the monopoly on this useful herb. A member of the mint family, the leaves of the catnip yield a pleasing and useful tea. It was much appreciated in England before the introduction of Asian teas and was also used by the Native Americans. It is therapeutic as an inducer of perspiration in cases of fever, as a carminative, and as a relaxant and sleep inducer. Catnip tea is said to work wonders with colicky infants; it is soothing and quieting and may save mothers some sleepless nights. For you or your child, steep 1 teaspoon dried or fresh crushed catnip leaves in 2 cups boiling water, and reap the calming benefits.

CAYENNE PEPPER   This red spice comes from bushy tropical pepper plants of the genus *Capsicum*—a completely different species from the black-pepper-producing vine, *Piper nigrum*. Extremely useful as a stimulant, it gives tone to the circulation and heals lacerations. It will even warm your feet if you sprinkle a little on the bottom of your socks!

Add cayenne to any dish that needs a lift—fish sauce, cream soup, eggs, cheese dishes. Remember that heat brings out the hot flavor, so stir a little before you taste. Cayenne differs in degree of hotness, depending on the source; certain imported types are generally more potent than domestic brands.

WELSH RAREBIT

   3 tablespoons butter
   1 pound cheddar cheese (sharp or mild, or combination of the two), cubed
   ½ cup quality beer
   ¼ teaspoon dry mustard
   ⅛ teaspoon cayenne pepper
   1 egg, beaten
   Salt to taste

- Melt the butter in the top of a double boiler. Add the cubed cheese and cook until just melted. Add beer slowly, then spices, and then the beaten egg a little at a time. Taste and add salt if necessary.
- Serve hot over whole wheat toast. This old-time English recipe is the ultimate in comfort food, enjoy!
- Serves two generously.

CELERY FLAKES   Dehydrated celery leaves, called flakes, can be used in much the same manner as dried parsley, particularly in cream sauces and soups.

CELERY SALT   The mineral content of celery is very high, and when the vegetable is dehydrated it produces a nutritious salty seasoning that tastes like—celery! Sprinkle on all foods that ask for this flavorful touch.

CELERY SEED   This aromatic celery-tasting seed can be used to flavor soups and cream or cottage cheese. A tea made from the seeds (1 teaspoon to 1 cup boiling water) is said to be of therapeutic value in the treatment of rheumatism, flatulence, and to stimulate the appetite.

CEREAL   Commercial cereals are devitalized to the point of absurdity. *Always* use whole grain cereals—unpopped, unpuffed, and un-sugarcoated. They will give you your money's worth as well as your health's worth, for straight untreated grains are far less expensive pound for pound than their "enriched" processed counterparts.

Whole grain non-precooked cereals do take longer to prepare; on early winter mornings this is not always desirable. Here are a few short cuts: Use the finer ground cereals (such as buckwheat grits instead of buckwheat groats, finely ground steel-cut oats instead of coarsely ground, cracked wheat instead of whole kernel wheat); what you lose in texture you will gain in cooking time. Or use the thermos jar method: In the evening, before bed, fill a wide-mouthed thermos with hot water; let it stand while cooking ½ cup whole grain in 2 cups boiling water for a couple of minutes; then pour the water out of the thermos and pour in the cereal and its cooking water. Add ½ cup raisins or currants if you like; close tightly and lay thermos on its side. Wake up to steaming hot cereal, ready to eat instantly with honey and cream.

Toasted granola–type whole grain cereals are popular items on the health market. They can be delicious as an instant cereal or dry snack; however, if you have any digestive or intestinal problems, be sure to soak them for 10–15 minutes before eating. Bircher-muesli, the original "health" cereal, has the nutritional advantage of being made of uncooked grain. When using packaged muesli, again presoak, if necessary, to soften grain and rocklike raisins. But why not make your own granola and muesli?

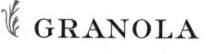 GRANOLA

> 6 cups oat flakes
> 1 cup sesame seeds, raw
> 1 cup wheat germ, raw
> Pinch of sea salt
> ⅓ cup pressed oil
> ⅔ cup honey

OPTIONAL:
> ½ cup shredded coconut
> 1 cup raw peanuts
> 1 cup raisins

- ❧ Preheat oven to 300 degrees.
- ❧ Mix together all ingredients (except raisins) with a wooden spoon, and spread out on a baking sheet. Bake, stirring every 10 minutes, until light brown—about 30–40 minutes. While the granola cools, add raisins if desired.
- ❧ Store in a well-sealed container. Granola keeps well without refrigeration—so this recipe makes a goodly amount. If it becomes a little soggy after a while, simply re-crisp it in the oven.
- ❧ Makes about nine cups of granola.

🌿 MUESLI

>1 cup oat flakes
>1 cup milk
>1 tablespoon lemon juice
>3 tablespoons honey
>1 apple, grated
>1 tablespoon raisins
>1 tablespoon chopped hazelnuts

- ❧ Soak oat flakes in milk for 30 minutes. Add lemon juice, honey, grated apple (skin and all if it is organic), raisins, and nuts. Mix well.
- ❧ Serves three.
- ❧ *Note:* Any cereal flakes can substitute for the oats in muesli and granola: wheat, rye, barley, rice, soya, etc.

CHAMOMILE   An old favorite among herbs, chamomile was cherished by the ancient Egyptians, who claimed that its aromatic tea was a mild—but not to be disparaged!—elixir of youth. A more concrete value of this wildflower lies in its sedative power; brew yourself a cup of chamomile tea (1 teaspoon chamomile to 1 cup boiling water and steep 10 minutes) before going to bed, add a little honey, and sleep will find you with utmost speed! Even the illustrious young Peter Rabbit was sent to bed with a calming cup of chamomile after his adventures in Farmer MacGregor's garden.

The tea is calming for nervous conditions, for regulating menstruation, and alleviating cramps. It is soothing in instances of indigestion and neuralgia. Administer a mild dose of tea to infants for alleviating teething pains. A compress soaked in a strong solution of chamomile tea will ease irritation of inflamed areas of skin—you might try this for complexion problems. If you want to make your blond hair blonder, by all means try a chamomile rinse. It's very simple: Boil ½ ounce chamomile flowers in a pint of water for 20 minutes; strain and pour over hair after washing.

CHARCOAL   Charcoal has a remarkable ability to absorb fermenting gases and poisonous substances; it lends itself to many uses. Charcoal filters have been used for many years to draw out noxious substances from drinking water. Butter carefully packed in charcoal will keep for a year. A small bag of charcoal kept in the silverware drawer will absorb the sulfur gases that cause tarnish. In drawers, closets, and poorly ventilated rooms a bag of charcoal pieces will absorb musty odors.

Medicinally, charcoal will alleviate gaseous conditions, heartburn, and dysentery. If administered immediately following accidental poisoning, it will help to draw some of the poison away from the body. (In case of poisoning, however, your first step, of course, is to call a doctor!) A poultice made of powdered charcoal can alleviate skin conditions—burns, bruises, inflammation of the eyes. Charcoal comes in powder and pill form and should be made of the finest soft woods.

CHEESE   All cheeses are made of coagulated milk, but the methods of aging cheese are so innumerable and the types of milk used so various, that we are faced in our lifetimes with the happy prospect of savoring hundreds upon hundreds of deliciously different kinds of cheese.

The character of a cheese depends on whether cow, goat, sheep, or buffalo milk is used; on how much cream is added to or left out of the milk; on what kind of coagulator is used (nowadays this is usually rennin, an enzyme taken from the stomach of a calf, but in times gone by vinegar, fig juice, and decoctions of thistle tops and artichoke flowers were also used); and on how long the cheese is aged (this can be anywhere from two days to two years). Spices, wines, or herbs may be added to lend distinctive flavor.

Cheese making used to be a local farmhouse activity. Farmer Brown's cheese would be different from neighbor Jones's, because their cows grazed on opposite sides of the dirt road. Today, however, cheese markets are monopolized and degraded by giant concerns. We find "Swiss" cheese made in Wisconsin and "Italian fontina" made in Sweden. Inevitably taste and quality suffer.

And then there are the additives (not to mention pesticide residues, an enormous problem)—stabilizers, emulsifiers, dyes, bleaches, preservatives. Ever wonder why cream cheese and cottage cheese will last for six weeks in your refrigerator? Try making your own (see recipes below), and you will find that if the delicious stuff is not eaten in three days or so, it starts to ferment and then to mold—that is a healthy sign! Always rejoice if you find a forgotten piece of cheese that has gone moldy on you; that means it is alive. There are Wisconsin "Swiss" cheeses that can sit looking beautiful in the icebox for months with absolutely no change in appearance or flavor—just imagine the unwholesome chemicals that must be used to produce such an unnatural state of affairs.

Try to buy traditionally made regional cheeses. There are still true Vermont cheddars and smoked Oregon Tillamooks and homemade Italian ricottas around, and the recent rebirth in the United State of fine cheeses produced by small family-run farms has made it possible to experience the truly delectable nature of a fine, fresh cheese. Try to find cheese made from the milk of organically raised cows, and if possible, from certified raw milk. Then you will enjoy the full benefits of the calcium and protein with which cheese abounds, without fear of pesticide contamination.

Never resort to processed cheese. It is prepared from ground-up low-quality cheese and made smooth or spreadable by the addition of harmful emulsifiers. There are a myriad of excellent European cheeses available to us, but they too have their problems with pesticide residues and additives. Whether native or foreign, try to buy cheese that you can watch being cut from its original large piece; often additives are listed on a large round of cheese but omitted when it is repackaged in small pieces.

Here are some recipes for naturally curdled cheeses that can easily be made at home. They will show you what good fresh cheese should taste like.

❦ CREAM CHEESE

- ❧ Let a pint of heavy cream sour at room temperature. This will take about 2 days. Pour into a cheesecloth bag and let it drain. When solid, refrigerate.

❦ COTTAGE CHEESE

- ❧ Heat 2 quarts milk in a large enamel pot until barely lukewarm. Place covered in a warm spot—in the sun in summer, or in the stove in winter (warm the oven every once in a while to keep the temperature at about 85 degrees).
- ❧ In 1 or 2 days the curd will have risen to the top and the whey will be on the

bottom. Put curd in a colander lined with a piece of cheesecloth, drain, then draw up cloth and squeeze out as much liquid as possible. This can be flavored with salt, caraway seeds, chopped chives, etc.

🐦 If a harder cheese is desired, more like mozzarella, keep the milk at a slightly higher temperature—about 115 degrees.

🐦 Makes about 14 ounces of cheese.

These cheeses can be used to make:

🌿 COEUR A LA CRÈME

½ cup cottage cheese

½ cup cream cheese

½ cup heavy cream

¼ cup raw sugar

1 tablespoon kirsch (or ¼ teaspoon vanilla)

🐦 Cream all together. Press into traditional heart-shaped baskets or porcelain molds, lined with cheesecloth. Chill for 2 hours. Unmold and serve with jam or fresh fruit.

🐦 Serves four.

🌿 TOMATO AND CHEESE PIE

1 piecrust (see piecrust recipe in book)

2 large onions, thinly sliced

¾ tablespoon fresh rosemary, chopped

4 tablespoons butter

3 large tomatoes

3 tablespoons olive oil

Salt and pepper to taste

¾ cup freshly grated Parmesan cheese

10 ounces mozzarella cheese, sliced into ¼-inch slices

1 (2-ounce) tin flat anchovy filets, rinsed and patted dry with
      paper towel (reserve oil)

8 black olives (preferably oil-cured), pitted, sliced in half

🐦 Preheat oven to 350 degrees.

🐦 Sauté onions and rosemary in the butter until soft and lightly colored, set aside.

- Dip tomatoes in boiling water for 1 minute. Remove and slip skins off. Cut in half horizontally and squeeze to remove seeds. Chop. Cook tomatoes in olive oil over moderate heat until they are soft and almost all the liquid is gone. Season with salt and pepper.
- Sprinkle grated cheese into the pie shell. Spoon cooked onions onto it. Spread tomatoes over the onions. Layer the mozzarella on the onions and tomatoes. Arrange anchovy filets in a lattice over the cheese. Dip olive halves in anchovy oil and place in the lattice openings.
- Bake for 30 minutes.
- Serves four to six.

CHERRY, DRIED   The cherry is said to be effective in the treatment of gout and arthritis and as such has taken its stand on dried food shelves. It is high in vitamin C and iron; syrup made from the dried or fresh fruit is a time-honored cough remedy.

CHERRY BARK TEA   The dried inner bark of the North American wild cherry tree is used to make this tea. It is useful in the treatment of mucous coughs and asthma and is said to strengthen the stomach. To brew, steep 1 teaspoon bark in 1 cup of boiling water for 3–5 minutes.

CHERVIL   A delicate herb for the educated palate, this fernlike leaf of the carrot family lends sweet fragrance to salads, cream soups, *sauce béarnaise*, and *aux fines herbes*. Planted in fall and harvested in spring, chervil has long been used as a spring tonic; it is said to have blood-cleansing and diuretic qualities. Use it generously in the kitchen—it never overpowers but rather enhances other herbal flavors.

CHESTNUT   Chestnuts have graced the tables of Europe for centuries in the widest variety of forms, from the exalted *marron glacé* to the common porridge. The chestnut is rich in potassium and contains good quantities of sodium and magnesium. It can be used as a potato substitute, for unlike other nuts, the chestnut is predominantly starchy rather than oily.

To prepare fresh chestnuts for cooking: With a sharp knife cut two slits in a cross form on the nut; bake in a hot oven until they split; peel (if your mouth is watering, stop here—they're delicious!). To prepare dried chestnuts for cooking: Soak overnight in water; if they are to be cooked in ample water an hour or more, presoaking is unnecessary.

CHESTNUT RICE

2½ cups water

1½ teaspoons salt

1 cup brown rice

½ cup dried chestnuts

2 chopped scallions (or 1 medium onion)

2 tablespoons butter

Bring salted water to boil. Add rice so slowly that water does not stop boiling. Add dried chestnuts. Cover tightly and simmer about 45 minutes, or until water is absorbed and rice is fluffy. Meanwhile sauté chopped scallions in butter. When chestnut rice is ready, toss with scallion butter and serve.

Serves four.

CHICKPEA　The curious name that English has fastened to this Asiatic legume is merely a phonetic adaptation of the original Latin *Cicer* and the French *pois chiche*—there is truly nothing to do with young chickens here! Chickpeas grow one or two to the pod and are a valuable food, rich in calcium, potassium, sodium, iron, phosphorus, and protein. In dry form they must be soaked in water overnight and then simmered for 3 hours (or until tender) before serving.

Chickpeas and rice with a little rosemary, butter, salt, and pepper make a delicious dish; add some chicken broth and you will have transformed this into a tasty soup. Cooled and seasoned with salad dressing, chickpeas make a refreshing summer salad or all-season antipasto. Here follows a zestful dip for bread or crackers—though you may end up eating it by the spoonful—a version of the Middle Eastern hummus.

CHICKPEA PURÉE (HUMMUS)

2 cups chickpeas, soaked and cooked

½ cup olive or sesame seed oil

⅓ cup fresh lemon juice

3 cloves garlic, finely chopped

½ teaspoon salt

½ cup sesame tahini

To prepare in blender: Put all ingredients in a blender except chickpeas; blend well. Slowly add chickpeas; blend to a smooth paste. If too thick, add a little water.

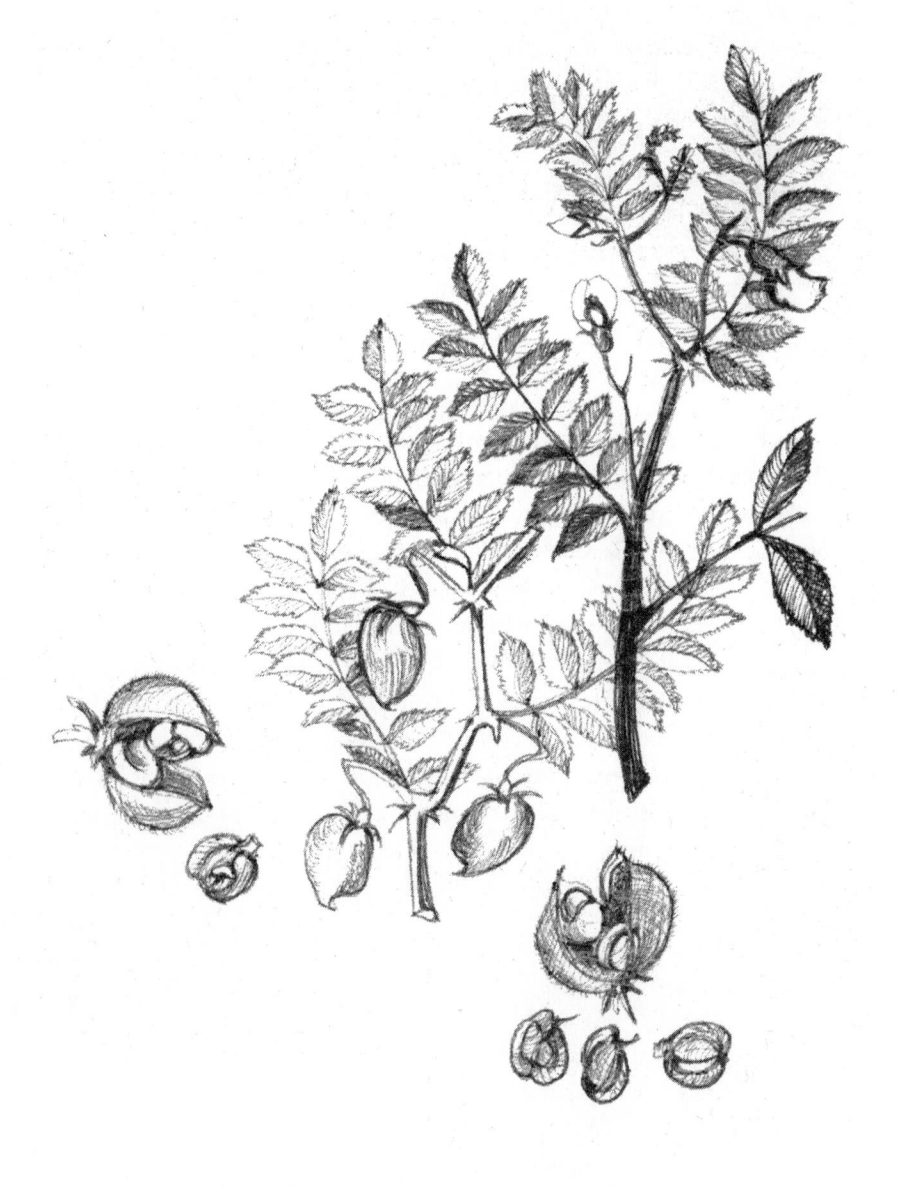

CHICKPEA
Plant—½ size
Seeds—life size

THE DICTIONARY OF WHOLESOME FOODS

- If you have no blender, mash the chickpeas thoroughly and mix in the other ingredients well. Serve cold.
- Serves four.

❦ CHICKPEA AND TOMATO SOUP

    2 large onions, chopped
    4 cloves garlic, chopped
    1 heaping tablespoon fresh rosemary, chopped
    1 (35 ounce) can Italian tomatoes, chopped
    2 (9.5 ounce) cans chickpeas
    Salt and pepper

- Sauté onions, garlic, and rosemary in olive oil until golden. Add tomatoes and juice; add one can of chickpeas, salt, and pepper. Cook 10 minutes. Purée. Add other can of chickpeas. Purée the soup again, or roughly chop if you prefer it chunky. If too thick, add vegetable or chicken broth.
- Serve hot or cold, with a spoonful of yogurt in the middle and a sprig of rosemary.
- Serves four.

CHICORY   Where would the coffee of France and New Orleans be without its chicory? For it is the mixture of the roasted chicory root with the coffee bean that yields the distinctive brew of these areas. (Purist coffee lovers might call this adulteration rather than mixture.)

Chicory is a wild plant that is often brought under cultivation (more in Europe than in the United States); its delicate blue flowers close at night and then open again with clocklike regularity in the morning hours. The plant shares many of the medicinal and culinary uses of its relative the dandelion. Its tasty bitter leaves act as a stimulant to the appetite and digestion and can be eaten raw in salad or cooked as a vegetable. The leaves can also be chopped and brewed as a tea that is useful for liver ailments, gout, and rheumatism. The chicory root, ground and roasted, is used as a coffee substitute, and when combined with coffee is said to counteract its stimulating effects.

CHIVES   This most refined member of the onion family is mild in taste, has a stimulating effect on the appetite, and has none of the digestion-disturbing tendencies of the onion. The leaves are the most used part of the plant (when growing your own, do not encourage the beautiful blue flowers; they toughen the herb, although the tiny bulbs can be pickled as an unusual delicacy). Frozen chives should be reconstituted in a little water before using. Add this chopped greenery to vichyssoise, salads, and omelets; simultaneously you will be adding good supplies of vitamins A and C and potassium to your diet.

CHLORELLA This freshwater algae has a higher chlorophyll content than any other plant, including alfalfa. Considered by many to be useful in detoxifying the body, chlorella is said to absorb toxins in the body, remove alcohol from the liver, treat viral and bacterial infections, and relieve constipation. Chlorella can also be mixed with water to form a paste that can be applied topically to aid in healing cuts and wounds.

Chlorella contains comparable nutrients to that of spirulina—high in protein, amino acids, and beta-carotene—but has twice the amount of chlorophyll and nucleic acid. Chlorella is more difficult to harvest and process than other blue-green algae, which drives up the price of chlorella considerably. However, due to its high nutrient content, less is needed to experience results. Chlorella is available in powder and capsule form.

CINNAMON True cinnamon is cultivated in much of the tropical world, including South America, the Pacific, Africa, and tropical Asia. The bark is cut off the cinnamon tree in long strips and slowly dried into "quills"—those long, curling, tubular cinnamon sticks with which we are familiar. Often used to adulterate ground cinnamon is "cassia," or Chinese cinnamon, which is more easily and widely cultivated (and therefore cheaper) and has a taste very similar to real cinnamon, though more pungent and less delicate. So if you want to be sure of your cinnamon, buy it in stick form.

Cinnamon was highly prized in ancient times as a perfume, medicine, preservative, and flavoring spice; small quantities of the precious quills were considered fit gifts for kings. The Arabs, who first brought cinnamon to the West, shrouded its origins in grotesque mysteries to frighten off rival traders. As you stir your espresso with a cinnamon quill and nibble on a cinnamon cookie, imagine yourself the envy of ancient potentates and bedaggered Arabs.

CARROT CAKE WITH CREAM CHEESE FROSTING

    2 cups whole wheat pastry flour
    2 teaspoons baking soda
    1 teaspoon salt
    2 teaspoons cinnamon
    ¼ cup vegetable oil (preferably pressed oil)
    ¼ cup honey
    4 eggs, well beaten
    3½ cups grated carrots

- Preheat oven to 350 degrees. Oil and flour two 8-inch layer pans or one 8-inch springform pan.
- Sift together the flour, soda, salt, and cinnamon. Stir in oil and honey, and then the well-beaten eggs. Mix in the grated carrots.
- Pour batter in prepared pans and bake for 35 minutes. Remove from pans and cool on a cake rack while you prepare the cream cheese frosting below—also delicious unfrosted.

CREAM CHEESE FROSTING:
    8 ounces cream cheese
    8 tablespoons (1 stick) unsalted butter
    3 cups powdered sugar

- Have cream cheese and butter at room temperature. Cream together, using a spoon or fingers. Add powdered sugar until desired consistency is reached. Makes enough frosting for a two-layer cake.

CLOVE   The dried flower buds of the large evergreen clove tree form this nail-shaped spice. The name "clove" is derived from the French *clou*, meaning nail. Originally native to the Molucca (or Spice) Islands, the clove tree was smuggled out to other islands with intricate subterfuge by spice-hungry colonialist nations.

The clove is now used primarily as a culinary spice, excellent for adding flavor to baked goods and spiced drinks. But its uses are far more varied. To chew a clove sweetens the breath, and ancient Chinese officials were once allowed to approach their monarch only when holding cloves in their mouths. A few cloves brewed with tea add enticing flavor, as well as giving a carminative effect to the tea. In a container of water set on a warm stove, they will deodorize a room.

Mulled wine flavored with cloves offers a more exciting way to aid the digestion than most commercial concoctions. Clove oil is a natural pain reliever and can be used to relieve toothaches. As a tincture, clove is said to be effective in the treatment of athlete's foot and well as other fungal infections.

In the kitchen, use cloves sparingly, for their flavor is heavy. Try tossing an onion studded with a few cloves into your next pot of stew or rice.

On rainy autumn days your children might enjoy the sweet-smelling activity of pomander-ball making; they will be ready in time for the holidays.

POMANDER BALLS

Oranges, thin-skinned
Cloves aplenty
Cinnamon, powdered

- Make sure the oranges are a thin-skinned variety, or there will be sore fingers at the end of this game. For added protection, Band-Aids can be placed for padding on appropriate fingers—what child will not love an excuse for a Band-Aid!
- Stud each orange all over with cloves, pushing them right in up to their tops. Roll studded oranges in powdered cinnamon, and pat on a heavy coating. Wrap each fruit in tissue paper, place in a cupboard or dark, cool place, and cure it for about six weeks. Then shake off excess cinnamon and the pomanders are ready to impart their sweet smell to closets and cupboards.

COCONUT, SHREDDED   The tall, slender coconut tree lends itself to myriad uses. Its trunk is used for timber, its flower spathes for crude sugar and toddy and arrack liquor, its leaves for roofing and basket weaving, its husk for rope making, its shells for drinking vessels, and its kernels for oil and coconut milk and "meat." Coconut palms are found growing in tropical countries throughout the world, particularly on seacoasts, for the rounded, triangular-shaped coconut is easily carried by ocean currents to far-off shores.

Shredded coconut is made from the meat of the coconut, the white inner lining of the kernel. It is used primarily in the preparation of desserts, for its sweet nutty flavor. Commercially you will find it in both moist and dry form; moist coconut has more unpleasant additives than the dry, but both are likely to be sweetened with unhealthful sugar—which is foolishness, for coconut is loaded with its own valuable natural sugar. So buy it desiccated and without additives at

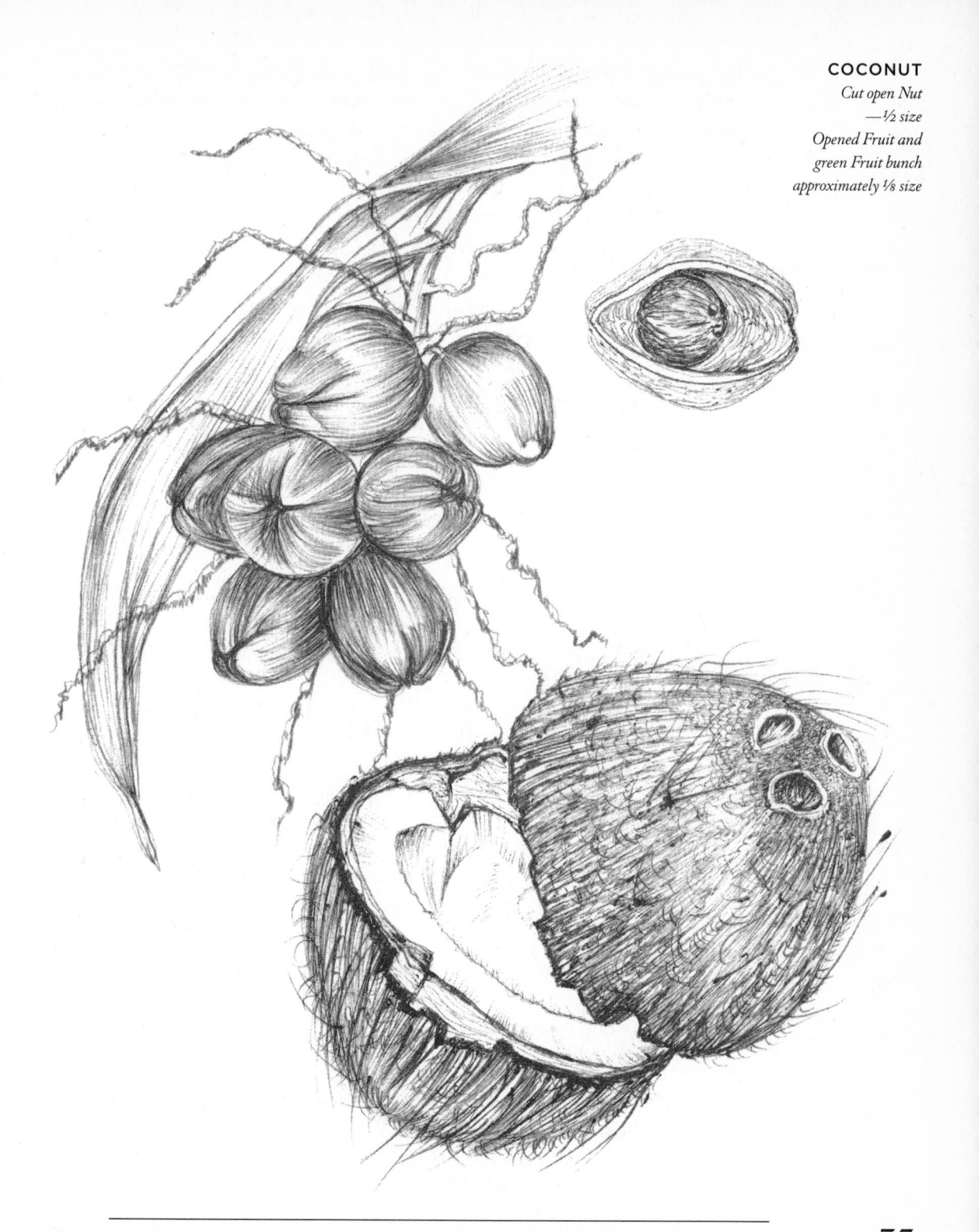

COCONUT
Cut open Nut
—½ size
Opened Fruit and
green Fruit bunch
approximately ⅛ size

your health food store. Or if you are handy with a knife and steady of arm, prepare your own—it will be naturally moist, utterly delicious, and very economical.

Coconut meat will add protein, potassium, phosphorus, magnesium, and a touch of iodine to your desserts. It is low in carbohydrates and contains less fat than most other nuts.

FRESH SHREDDED COCONUT

If you can hear the milk lapping inside the coconut when you shake it, it is ripe and ready. Pierce the "eyes" of the coconut with a screwdriver and drain out the milk (you can drink this on the spot, or use it as liquid in any dessert recipe— it is very nutritious). Put coconut in a 400-degree oven for 15–20 minutes. Remove it from the oven and immediately give coconut a sharp blow with a hammer, and the shell will fall away from the meat. Trim off the dark skin. Grind the white meat in a blender. Keep it moist in a jar in the refrigerator; it will stay fresh for about two weeks. Or dry it slowly in the oven and it will not have to be refrigerated.

COCONUT UPSIDE-DOWN CAKE

　　　6 tablespoons butter
　　　1/2 cup raw or brown sugar
　　　1 1/2 cups fresh shredded coconut (or desiccated coconut plus
　　　　　2 tablespoons water)

BATTER:

　　　1 1/2 cups whole wheat pastry flour
　　　2 1/2 teaspoons baking powder
　　　1/2 teaspoon salt
　　　8 tablespoons (1 stick) butter
　　　3/4 cup sugar (preferably raw sugar)
　　　1 egg plus 1 egg yolk, well beaten
　　　1/2 teaspoon vanilla extract
　　　1/2 cup coconut (or dairy) milk

In a flat-bottomed 8-inch iron skillet, melt 6 tablespoons butter, 1/2 cup sugar. Add 1 1/2 cups fresh shredded coconut (or desiccated coconut plus 2 tablespoons water). In a large bowl sift flour, baking powder, and salt three times. Cream 8 tablespoons butter, 3/4 cup sugar, eggs, and vanilla. Mix half of creamed mixture into dry ingredients, then half of the liquid, then the other half of creamed mixture, then the last half of liquid. Do not overmix.

- Pour into skillet on top of coconut. Bake at 350 degrees for about 35 minutes. Remove from the oven, loosen the sides with a knife; immediately flip over onto a cake platter. Serve warm or cool.
- Serves six to eight.

COCONUT OIL   Coconut oil, extracted from the copra or dried meat of the coconut kernel, is one of the most highly saturated of all vegetable oils. Note that many of the so-called high in unsaturates margarines use coconut oil as a hardening agent—an oil that is more saturated than butter itself!

Although coconut oil can be used for cooking purposes, it is most widely used in the manufacture of cosmetics. It is also said to be useful in mitigating muscular aches when massaged into the affected area, and in preventing stretch marks during pregnancy.

COFFEE SUBSTITUTES   There was an anti-coffee bandwagon long before health foodists appeared on the scene. When early Muslims began using coffee as a "devotional anti-soporific" to see them through lengthy religious services, they stirred up fierce controversy with orthodox priests, who regarded coffee as a forbidden intoxicant. Later, in the sixteenth century, the establishment of coffeehouses in Constantinople excited the wrath of the ecclesiastics, for they cut down on church attendance. In England, the first coffeehouses were established in the seventeenth century and aroused the hostility of King Charles II himself, who claimed that they were a "disturbance to the peace and quiet of the nation" and harbored undesirable dissidents.

These rocky times passed, however. The raising of coffee became an enormously lucrative enterprise and spread from its native Abyssinia to all tropical parts of the world. The roasted seeds of the red fruit of the coffee plant began to be held in high regard as an alleviator of fatigue and sustainer of strength under stress.

Not until the twentieth century has coffee been strongly attacked on purely dietary grounds. Now we hear that it raises the blood sugar level of the body at an alarming rate, that it aggravates ulcers and heart conditions, that it leads to vitamin B deficiency, that it is habit-forming, that mixed with cream it is bad for the digestion, that it is full of harmful caffeine and tannic acid … and so we have the coffee substitutes: roasted grains, figs, beans, dandelion roots, chicory roots. No one will argue that the substitutes are indeed more healthful than coffee, and there are those who may find them toothsome. The only trouble is, they just don't taste much like coffee.

If you persist in sticking with the real thing, you can palliate the bad effects somewhat by brewing coffee with the filter or espresso methods, which are said to release less tannic acid into your cup. Also, a snack of sunflower seeds (or other protein food) may help to prolong the "high" you get from your cup of coffee, by shoring it up with a real energy source. Be sure to resolutely stick to organic, shade-grown coffee beans that have been purchased under fair trade; to do otherwise is to risk not only your own health but the health and well-being of the workers on coffee plantations.

COLTSFOOT   The yellow-flowered coltsfoot (*Tussilago farfara*), whose leaves are shaped like the hoof of a colt, may be found growing in moist soils and alongside streams in Europe, Canada, and the northeastern United States. It is most conspicuous in early spring, when its dandelion-like flowers appear, and can quickly move to overrun a garden. Although all parts of the plant possess some medicinal qualities, it is the fragrant leaves that are used for teas and poultices. As a tea or tincture, coltsfoot is high in vitamin C, and is used to allay coughing; as an expectorant it helps to clean the respiratory tract. A cloth moistened in coltsfoot tea and applied to the throat or chest will relieve those areas of congestion. To prepare coltsfoot tea, steep 1 teaspoon leaves in 1 cup boiling water for 30 minutes. Pregnant and nursing women should avoid this herb; coltsfoot should not be used for extended periods of time.

COMFREY   Knitbone, boneset, healing herb—these popular names for comfrey are indicative of its extraordinary medicinal qualities. It is particularly well known for its ability to speed the healing of fractured and broken bones; either the roots or the leaves are pounded into a mucilaginous mass and applied as a poultice to the injured area, and the tea is taken internally. Comfrey poultices have been said to effect wondrous cures of malignant ulcers; again tea from either root or leaf is taken conjointly, internally. Comfrey tea is also useful in the treatment of chest disorders and tuberculosis, internal ulcers, and diarrhea. To prepare the tea, steep 1 teaspoon leaves or root in 1 cup boiling water for 30 minutes.

Comfrey (Symphytum officinale) grows wild in many parts of the world, including North America. It is also easily cultivated as a garden plant.

CONGEE   A traditional breakfast food in China, congee is made by simmering rice with five times its amount in water. The result is a thin, nutritional porridge. Congee can be simmered from half an hour to five or six hours, with the longer duration producing the more powerful congee. Reputed to soothe digestion and tonify the blood, congee can be easily made at home and is a perfect first food for those recovering from the stomach flu. Congee is a soothing food for the chronically ill and is said to increase the milk flow in nursing mothers. The liquid from the congee can be poured off and administered to infants, as well as those who are unable to hold down solid food.

CORIANDER   The name of this aromatic spice gives no indication of its culinary potential—"coriander" is derived from the Greek *coris*, an ill-smelling bug whose odor was thought to be similar to that of fresh coriander seed. Only when dried does the seed assume the goodly character that lends itself so well to dessert making, curries, and many South American dishes. Tea made from the crushed seeds is carminative; the flavorful seeds can also be mixed with herbs and spices whose taste alone might be unpalatable.

Coriander leaves, also known as cilantro, which look rather like those of the carrot, add unusual seasoning to salads and soups—no problem with odors here, for the leaves are delicious fresh or dried.

CORN, FLAKED   Do not confuse this with the cornflake of supermarket breakfast cereal notoriety. This is the crushed whole kernel of corn, with all its natural goodness intact. Unlike most whole flaked grains, which have only to be soaked before eating, these corn flakes require light cooking. See also *Cornmeal*.

CORN FLOUR   Finely ground kernels of corn yield a flour—white, yellow, or (in the southwest United States) blue, depending on the type of corn used—that has a distinctive corn taste, but does not have the mealy texture one usually associates with ground corn products. It is good added to soups and stews as a thickener and can be substituted in bread recipes for a portion of wheat flour. If you feel adventurous, try using it instead of meal in cornmeal recipes—you will be inventing a new dish all your own, and one bound to taste good. See also *Cornmeal*.

CORN GRITS   Coarser in grind than cornmeal, but finer than flaked corn, these grits make a grand breakfast cereal. They are far more nutritious than the traditional white hominy grits, which are dehulled and degermed. Corn grits can also be used for making a more textured polenta or cornmeal mush. See also *Cornmeal*.

CORN KERNEL, DRIED   Dried corn kernels are for those who prefer to grind their own meal....And that cannot be beat! These kernels are not meant for cooking whole, as they take forever and a day to soften. See also *Cornmeal.*

CORN OIL   One of the most unsaturated of vegetable oils, this oil is ideal for all types of cooking and can also be used for salad dressings. Its high smoke point makes corn oil ideal for frying. Be sure to buy it in as unprocessed a state as possible. Aim for crude pressed corn oil, though it is hard to find. A darker color will be one indication that the oil contains more of its natural qualities.

CORN-SILK TEA   Fresh or dried corn silk, steeped 1 teaspoon to a cup of boiling water, is said to be beneficial for kidney and bladder ailments, to ease water retention, and for treating urinary tract infections.

CORNMEAL   Controversy has long waged over the origins of the genus *Zea mays,* or maize—or if you will, common corn. There are those who assert that it is strictly American in origin; certainly the Native Americans were master corn cultivators long before Europeans set foot on these shores. Others claim that corn reached Europe from the East with the Arab invasions into Spain in the thirteenth century. In Italy, where cornmeal cookery has attained a fine art, the name for corn is *granturco*—Turkish grain—which certainly points to an Eastern origin.

Well, East or West, it is a superb food! Nutritionally it contains less protein and niacin than other grains, but unless your diet consists of absolutely nothing but refined cornmeal, your chances of getting pellagra—that old bugbear of cornmeal—are entirely nil. White cornmeal is milled from white corn and is said by some connoisseurs to have a more sophisticated flavor and smoother texture than meal from yellow corn. Yellow cornmeal, on the other hand, has a fuller taste and is more nutritious, for it contains carotene, which is converted by the body into vitamin A.

Never buy degerminated, overmilled, overheated, synthetic-vitamin-enriched commercial cornmeal—it has little health value and even less taste. Among properly milled whole kernel meals, flavor will vary depending on the type of corn used; buy in small quantities until you find the taste that pleases you. Texture is also a variant; some distributors label as "meal" grinds that are more like flour in fineness. What joy to be able to choose and not be constricted to standardized lifeless products!

❧ "FOOLPROOF" POLENTA

1 cup polenta (cornmeal)

1½ teaspoons salt

1 cup cold water

3 cups boiling water

- Mix polenta and salt. Add 1 cup of cold water and mix well. Add 3 cups of boiling water and stir together until thoroughly blended. Cook over boiling water in a double boiler. Cook for 20 minutes, or until soft, stirring occasionally.
- You may serve plain, or you may add 2–3 tablespoons of butter and ¼ cup grated Parmesan cheese. Mix together and serve as is or topped with fresh tomato sauce or stir-fried mushrooms.
- Serves four.

COSMETICS Now that "natural" and "organic" cosmetics are readily available on the market, it is possible to spend unprecedented amounts of money in order to moisturize, smooth, and otherwise beautify the face and body, all the while having a clear conscience that we are not polluting our bodies with mysterious and unidentifiable ingredients. The choices are many and the results often too obscure or subtle to notice, so while you are shopping around for the perfect solution to your skin and hair needs, make do with these safe and sure (and inexpensive) home treatments and remedies for skin health and safety:

ALOE A native to Africa, the beautiful aloe is a desert plant belonging to the lily family, which has earned it the alternate title of "Lily of the Desert." Aloe has been used for its healing properties for thousands of years, and continues to be used by those who are aware of its beneficial properties and myriad uses. Even those with a brown thumb should consider growing an aloe plant at home. Aloe is strikingly easy to grow. After all, this is a desert plant and it needs very little attention in order to flourish. It is well worth having fresh aloe leaves on hand to treat burns and cuts.

Inside of the plant is a mucilaginous gel that absorbs into the skin and provides a protective coating that both expedites healing and provides relief from both pain and itching. Aloe vera is soothing to sunburns and can be kept in the refrigerator in order to provide instant cooling relief. Aloe vera is available in a food-grade form, which is the next best thing when applied topically (if fresh leaves are not available), as it is missing the perfumes and additives commonly used in store-bought aloe products. Apply food-grade aloe directly to the face in order to expedite the healing of acne and blemishes.

Food-grade aloe can be mixed with a glass of water and taken internally, where it is reputed to purify the blood and liver, cleanse the colon and intestines, and to soothe ulcers. Aloe vera is said to alkalize the digestive juices, a process that soothes indigestion; however, do not ingest the leaf of the aloe plant or apply to deep wounds, as this can actually delay healing time.

BENTONITE CLAY This healing clay, which is mined largely in Montana and Wyoming, is soft, fine, and odorless. Useful as a facemask to cleanse and tighten pores, bentonite clay can be mixed with water (for oily skin), milk (for normal skin), or heavy cream (for dry skin). Mix into a thick paste and apply to the face and neck, and allow to dry, then rinse. Bentonite clay is also available in a liquid form that can be taken internally and is said to absorb toxins and cleanse the intestinal tract.

JOJOBA OIL Gathered from the crushed bean of the jojoba shrub, jojoba oil is native to the Sonora Desert of northwestern Mexico, Arizona, and Southern California. This woody evergreen shrub can grow as tall as fifteen feet and has a life span of one to two hundred years. The jojoba shrub flowers in the spring, produces fruit by August, and then, as the green fruit dries in the desert heat, its outer skin shrivels and pulls back to expose a wrinkled brown soft-skin seed, referred to as a nut or bean. These nuts, which are about the size of an olive, contain an odorless vegetable-like oil with fantastic properties. It takes seventeen pounds of jojoba seeds (there are about 1,700 seeds in a pound) to produce one gallon of jojoba oil, which earns jojoba a rather high price on the shelves.

Native Americans have utilized jojoba oil for hundreds of years, using it to treat all sorts of conditions: sores, cuts, burns, and as a skin and scalp conditioner. One of the great benefits of jojoba oil is its stability. It does not go rancid, as it is not really an oil but a polyunsaturated liquid wax, similar to sperm whale oil—minus the scent. Jojoba oil is hypoallergenic, does not clog pores, and can be used directly on the face, body, and scalp and hair to soften skin, reduce stretch marks and wrinkles, and as a general healing agent.

For sensitive and troubled complexions, a few drops of jojoba oil rubbed onto the face after a shower can be far less catastrophic to the pores than any of those high-priced lotions available at the health food store. Just remember, a little bit goes a long way; just a few drops can be enough.

MANUKA OIL   The manuka tree flourishes across New Zealand. However, the variety that is said to be the most intensely medicinal is found on the East Cape. The essential oil of manuka is stored in the leaves and then extracted through steam distillation, a process that utilizes no chemicals and produces a pure and unadulterated product. Relatively new to the Western market, this healing oil has long been used by the native Maori of New Zealand. Manuka oil is known to have antibacterial, antifungal, anti-inflammatory, and antiviral properties and is available as a pure oil, diluted oil, cream, and soap. Manuka is said to be extremely effective in the treatment of athlete's foot and other fungal type infections, and can be applied topically for a variety of ills, including pimples, insect bites, canker and cold sores, eczema, head lice, ring worm, warts, and for muscular aches and pains. Manuka soap is said to aid in the reduction of foot and body odor as well as to help reduce skin outbreaks.

For aching muscles, mix about twenty drops of manuka oil into your massage oil of choice. For cold sores, apply undiluted oil 4–5 times per day. Two or three drops of undiluted oil can be gargled to treat a sore throat, and the diluted oil, or the cream, is said to be effective on infant cradle cap. Apply the undiluted oil directly to stubborn cases of athlete's foot, or for milder cases or as a preventive measure, use the cream. The undiluted oil is also said to be effective on strep and staph infections that are resistant to antibiotics. For staph, apply directly to the skin, and for strep, use as a gargle. The taste may not be enticing, but the results should make up for it.

PAPAYA, FRESH   Tired of spending large sums of money on high-end facial products? For a quality facial peel at a fraction of the price, reach for a fresh papaya instead! Mash about ¼ cup of papaya pulp and apply to the entire face and neck and around the eyes (though avoid getting the papaya in the eyes). Allow the pulp to remain on the face for 10–15 minutes, then rinse clean. This treatment will reduce fine wrinkles and give a fresh, taut glow to the skin. A mild stinging sensation is normal and a sign that the papaya is working its magic. Should the stinging turn to burning, then simply remove with fresh water.

TEA TREE OIL   The native peoples of Australia—the Aborigines—have long been aware of the incredible antiseptic and healing properties of tea tree oil. Antiviral, antifungal, anti-inflammatory, tea tree oil is one essential oil that no medicine cabinet can do without. Tea tree oil can be diluted with vegetable oil (try jojoba!) and administered to cuts, scrapes, and athlete's foot. Tea tree oil, as is evident by its powerful scent, is strong and should not be applied full-strength to the face. Instead, dilute with water or oil and apply directly to blemishes, or add a few drops to your favorite facemask to expedite healing.

Three or four drops can be added to the bath during a flu or cold for its calming and cleansing effects. Add four to six drops of tea tree oil to ¼ cup water for a topical antibacterial wash. Four to five drops of tea tree oil can be added to one tablespoon of warm olive oil and used as antiviral and antibacterial eardrops. Tea tree oil is a worthy investment, not just because of its myriad uses, but because a little bit goes such a long way. With only a few drops or so needed at any given time, the bottle will begin to get dusty long before it grows empty.

COUSCOUS   The basic dish of North African cuisine, couscous can be extremely intricate to prepare, or utterly simple, depending on your approach. This is a semolina made from hard durum wheat—rich in gluten and protein—coarsely ground, but finer than either bulgur or cracked wheat. The traditional manner of preparing couscous calls for a *couscousière*, a colander tightly fitted over a base pot; a meat stew is placed in the bottom, and the couscous goes in the colander top to cook in the steam of the stew.

Here is a simple dish that can be made with ordinary Western kitchen utensils. Perhaps it will inspire you to delve into the more complex aspects of traditional couscous preparation.

❦ COUSCOUS WITH SHRIMP

1 cup couscous
2 tablespoons butter
2 cups boiling water
1 pound shrimp, shelled and deveined
5 tablespoons butter
6 tablespoons soy sauce
1 tablespoon chopped fresh ginger

- Sauté couscous in 2 tablespoons butter for 1 minute; then add boiling water and simmer, while stirring, for about 3 minutes. Cover, and let sit for 15 minutes while you cook the shrimp.
- Sauté the shrimp in 5 tablespoons butter, soy sauce, and chopped ginger for approximately 5 minutes, depending on size of shrimp. When shrimp is cooked

(firm but tender), stir in the couscous. Serve this quick and delicious main course with a large fresh salad.

🐚 Serves four.

CRACKED WHEAT   See *Wheat, Cracked*.

CUMIN   Feeling squeamish? Take cumin with your bread or wine, prescribes Pliny. Cumin is also supposed to induce a pallid complexion, and Pliny tells of students who took cumin to achieve that "studious" look. This herbaceous annual is native to Egypt, but long ago spread to Mediterranean shores and is now cultivated worldwide. Cumin resembles caraway in appearance and taste—but it is more bitter. Widely used in Mexican chili powders and Indian curries, it can also be added to breads, cookies, rice, and creamed dishes for an interesting variation on the more familiar caraway flavor. Used for strengthening the digestion, cumin relieves flatulence and abdominal cramping.

CURRANT, DRIED   Currants grow on shrublike plants that flourish both in the wild and under cultivation. They are akin to gooseberries, and the small rather translucent berries can be of black, red, or white variety. When fresh, they are used for pies, jellies, and wines. The black currant is the most commonly cultivated, dried, and sold commercially.

Dried black currants are rich in iron and vitamin C, are neat to eat, and delicious, too. An interesting alternative to raisins, they are not as strong tasting. Substitute them in any recipe that calls for raisins; their smallness does not interfere with slicing bread and cutting cookies the way large raisins sometimes tend to do. The delicate flavor of currants lends itself to exotic recipes—such as spiced rice, stuffed mussels, or stuffed grape leaves.

🌱 RICE WITH CURRANTS AND NUTS

3 cups water (or broth)
1 teaspoon salt
1½ cups brown rice
3 tablespoons pignoli nuts
⅓ cup dried currants
2 tablespoons butter
¾ teaspoon ground allspice
¼ teaspoon ground cinnamon

- ❧ Bring salted water to boil; sprinkle in rice without stopping boiling. Cover and simmer.
- ❧ Gently sauté nuts and currants in the butter. After rice has cooked about 30 minutes, add sautéed nuts and currants with butter, allspice, and cinnamon. Continue cooking for about 15 minutes or until rice is tender and fluffy.
- ❧ Serves four.

CURRY POWDER   This Indian condiment is composed of a large and variable number of herbs and spices. A conservative tally of basic ingredients yields: red and black pepper, cardamom, cinnamon, coriander, cumin, fenugreek, garlic, ginger, mustard, turmeric, and poppy seed. Each brand of curry powder uses its own variation of the basic recipe, and the results in your cooking pot will range from fiery hot to merely spicy. Diehard curry enthusiasts grind their own powder from freshly obtained ingredients.

The flavor of curry blends well with any number of foods and need not be limited to traditional main dishes. A dash in your salad dressing, creamed soups, egg dishes, and melted butter for vegetables will add new life to a meal.

CURRIED CHICKEN BREASTS

4 pairs of chicken breasts, skinned and boned

Juice of 2 lemons

²/₃ cup unbleached flour

¼ teaspoon salt

2 teaspoons butter

2 teaspoons pressed vegetable oil

SAUCE:

2 tablespoons butter

³/₄ cup finely chopped onion

1 clove garlic, finely chopped

1 small cooking apple, cored and chopped (peel only if not organically grown)

3 tablespoons curry powder

2 tablespoons unbleached flour

2 cups chicken broth

½ cup cream or yogurt

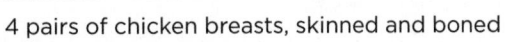

1 teaspoon lemon juice
1 tablespoon grated lemon rind
Pinch of cayenne pepper

🐦 If you bone your own chicken breasts (not difficult), use the bones to make the 2 cups of broth for sauce by simmering them for 3 hours in salted water. Cut boned and skinned chicken into small pieces, about 8 to each breast. Dip each piece in lemon juice, then in mixture of flour and salt. Warm 2 teaspoons butter and oil in a large skillet over medium heat, and brown chicken. Set aside in warm casserole.

🐦 In same pan, put the 2 tablespoons butter and sauté onion and garlic until transparent. Add apple and cook slowly until soft. Add curry powder and flour and make a smooth paste, adding broth a little at a time, and then the cream. Bring sauce to simmer, stirring all the while, then cook partially covered over very low heat for about 20 minutes. Add lemon juice and rind. Taste to see if sauce is spicy enough; if not, add a little cayenne pepper, but be careful not to overdo it—the taste of cayenne increases with cooking.

🐦 Pour sauce over chicken and stir to coat all pieces. Cook over low heat for 30 minutes. Serve immediately or set aside for later serving—even the next day.

🐦 Serve on a large bed of rice and with bowls of any of the following condiments:

> chutney
> chopped scallions
> diced avocado
> diced pineapple
> dried currants marinated in brandy
> shredded unsweetened coconut
> chopped salted peanuts, or chopped almonds
> hard-boiled eggs, finely chopped
> roasted pignoli nuts

🐦 Serves four royally.

KASHMIR LAMB CURRY

1 pound lean lamb cut into ½-inch pieces

2 cups plain yogurt

2 tablespoons curry powder (medium heat)

3 tablespoons oil

½ cup flaked or chopped blanched almonds

½ cup raisins

½ cup dried apricots

2 cloves garlic, sliced

2 onions, sliced

2 teaspoons lemon juice

¼ teaspoon salt

- Place meat, yogurt, and curry in a bowl. Stir, cover, and marinate for 3 hours in the refrigerator.
- Heat oil in a medium heavy-bottomed skillet. Sauté nuts until golden. Drain and set aside. Sauté raisins and apricots until plump. Drain and set aside. Sauté garlic and onions in remaining oil. Add meat and cook for 5 minutes. Add raisins, apricots, lemon juice, and salt. Cover and simmer until meat is tender, about 45–60 minutes. Sprinkle nuts on top.
- Serves four.
- *Note:* If you do not have time to marinate meat, follow recipe and when adding meat also add yogurt and curry. It works just fine.

D

DAIKON, DRIED   Daikon is a large white Japanese radish with a yin or acid tendency. When dried, it is long and stringlike and should be soaked for several hours before using. Chop it, sauté it, add salt and tamari sauce; also good with rice or other sautéed vegetables.

DANDELION   If you are accustomed to viewing the common dandelion as a garden nuisance—stop! This vitamin- and mineral-packed herb can be of great value to your health. Pick the plant in spring, when its leaves are young and tender; slice and cook the roots as a delicate vegetable, and use the leaves raw in salads for a zesty dish loaded with vitamin A. People on salt-restricted diets should go easy on the dandelions, however, for they contain large amounts of sodium. The yellow blossoms (if there are any left after your spring pickings) are traditionally used to make dandelion wine—a great favorite during Prohibition years in the United States.

You are most likely to find dandelion on the store shelf in the form of tea or as a coffee substitute. The tea, made from dried dandelion leaves, is considered an excellent blood cleanser and is helpful to digestion, the liver, and the gallbladder. Its chopped roasted roots are used as a coffee substitute, which unfortunately does not taste a great deal like coffee but possesses the same curative values as the tea.

DATE, DRIED   The tall and stately date palm has been cultivated in North Africa, the Middle East, and India since remote antiquity, and the date and its by-products have long been dietary staples in these areas. There the date is eaten fresh—an end-all of epicurean delights—pounded into cakes, ground to a flour, or its sap is rendered to sugar or made into various fermented beverages.

The Spaniards in the eighteenth century introduced the date palm into California, where it now thrives.

The date is rich in minerals such as potassium, magnesium, iron, and phosphorus, and in various B vitamins. It also has a very high sugar content. Dried dates make an extremely nutritious snack for children and are a great help in unseating the ubiquitous candy bar. They have a constipating tendency, the opposite of most other dried fruits. During the drying process, they are often treated with sulfuric acid; make sure to buy organically grown unsulfured dates.

For a special treat, try stuffing dates with nut butter or nutmeats—peanut butter and pecans go particularly well with dates.

DATE-NUT TARTS

Pastry for a double-crust pie

2 eggs

$\frac{1}{2}$ cup honey

$\frac{1}{4}$ teaspoon salt

$\frac{1}{2}$ cup finely chopped dates

$\frac{1}{2}$ cup chopped pecans or walnuts

1 teaspoon vanilla

4 tablespoons ($\frac{1}{2}$ stick) butter, melted

- Preheat oven to 350 degrees.
- Roll out pie dough on floured board and cut into rounds (a 4-inch-diameter piece of pastry will fit into a muffin form of 1¾-inch diameter). Press into muffin tins.
- Beat eggs well. Add honey and salt and beat vigorously. Stir in dates, nuts, vanilla, and butter. Fill each pastry cup about three-quarters full with this mixture. Bake 25 minutes or until browned and center is firm.
- Makes about one dozen.

DATE SUGAR   Date sugar can be made from the sap of the date palm. The date sugar that is most commonly seen in this country, however, is composed of ground dried dates. As dates have a sugar content of about 70 percent, these rich brown granules offer an excellent mineral-rich substitute for honey or cane sugar. See also *Date, Dried*.

DATE SYRUP   Date syrup is made of pulverized fresh dates. It makes a delicious and healthful sweet topping for yogurt, pancakes, waffles, and desserts. It can also be used in baking to replace sugar, honey, or molasses

DILL   Don't imprison this delightful herb in the pickle jar! Its uses as a tasty aromatic and a medicinal of long standing are far too various to accept such limitation. For hundreds of years dill tea has been used as a gentle sedative and as an aid to digestion. These attributes lend it power to calm nerves, hasten sleep, prevent nausea, increase the flow of a mother's milk, stop an infant's colic, even to chase away the hiccups. To make dill tea, steep ½ teaspoonful dill seed in a cup of hot water for 10 minutes; when administering to a baby, you can substitute milk for water.

In cooking, dill is just as useful. Dill salt, made from ground dill seeds, is a tasty salt substitute. Use either the seeds or the fresh or dried leaves sprinkled over salads, in cooking cabbage, in fish sauces (try dill with drawn butter) and broth, or mixed with cream cheese as a sandwich spread. Cucumbers and dill are a natural twosome; try serving this cucumber-yogurt soup with dill for a summer lunch with some good homemade bread beneath the cool shadows of a comfortable tree.

CUCUMBER-YOGURT SOUP WITH DILL

2 cucumbers
1 pint yogurt
Salt and pepper to taste
Dash of Worcestershire sauce
2 tablespoons chopped fresh dill
¼ teaspoon ground cumin

- Peel and finely chop cucumbers, or put through a blender. Put into soup tureen and add other ingredients. Mix well. Serve very cold with some extra dill sprinkled on top.
- Serves four.

🌾 SUMMER SQUASH RIBBON SALAD

5 tablespoons lemon juice

8 tablespoons olive oil

2–3 tablespoons fresh dill, chopped

Salt and pepper

1 shallot, finely chopped

2 medium yellow summer squash

2 medium zucchini

Beat lemon juice in olive oil. Add dill, salt and pepper, and shallot. Trim ends of the squash and slice in half. Using a wide peeler, place peeler at angle at the end of squash and zucchini and peel lengthwise, creating long, thin ribbons. Toss squash and zucchini ribbons with dressing.

Serves four to six.

DUKKA   Compromised of toasted nuts and seeds, dukka is an Egyptian spice that varies depending on the cook. Pistachio, hazelnut, chickpea, coriander, cumin, sesame, and thyme are all potential ingredients for dukka. The toasted ingredients are ground into a fine powder that can be sprinkled over salads, fish, or pasta. Dukka can be mixed with olive oil to form a paste for drizzling over warm breads.

DULSE   Extremely healthful and rich in organic iodine, fresh dulse (a dark red seaweed) is delicious in salads. Children in the Maritime Provinces of Canada chew on fresh dulse instead of candy. In health food stores dulse is found dried, and in this form it is quite leathery and tough; therefore it is usually used in cooking. Add it chopped to your soups, and forget the salt—dulse brings its own, in the most natural form possible.

DURUM WHEAT FLOUR   This is a hard, high-protein, high-gluten flour that is used for making pasta, semolina, and couscous. The grain is grown primarily in Russia, the United States, and Northern Africa.

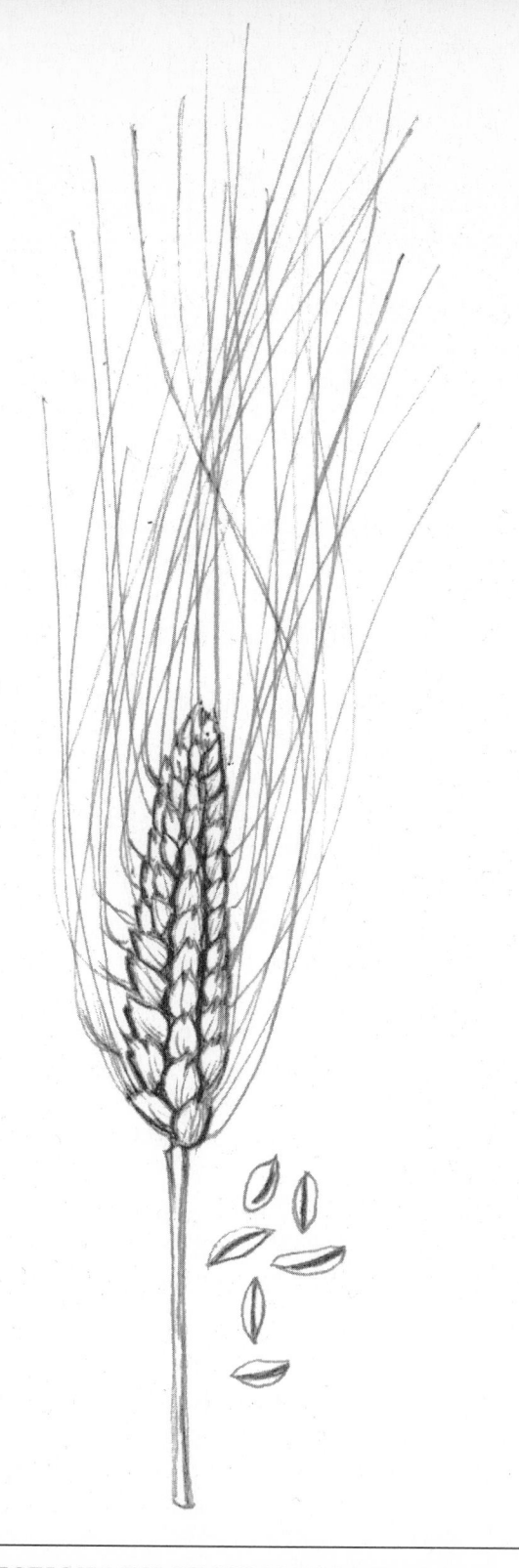

DURUM WHEAT
life size

E

ECHINACEA Also known as purple coneflower, besides being a beautiful addition to the garden, echinacea is one of the most popular herbal supplements on the market. Once used by Native Americans to treat snakebites, toothaches, sore throats, and coughs, echinacea has long been deemed an immune-boosting herb. Many studies have been done on echinacea, and it seems that it has the ability to stimulate the production of white blood cells, which fight infection and dispose of toxins in the body. It is suggested that echinacea be taken at intervals, a couple of weeks on and a couple of weeks off, as the body will eventually develop an insensitivity to the immune-boosting effects of this herb if taken continuously. While some claim echinacea to be an immune wonder herb, others seem to find it to be fairly innocuous. The best thing to do is give it a try and see how it works for your own particular immune system.

Echinacea, which grows wild on the midwestern prairies, is available in tinctures, capsule, and tea form. It can be taken to ward off illness as well as to shorten the duration of sickness once begun. Echinacea is safe for children and makes a great supplement during the cold and flu season.

EGGS, ORGANIC A good egg is hard to find! Today most hens live in overcrowded, disease-ridden, factory-type conditions—where a flock of 15,000 is considered small—without fresh air, natural light, or fresh food. They are fed antibiotics, Methedrine, tranquilizers, chemicals to make the yolk appear more yellow, and additives to make the shell harder.

How does one find eggs from chickens whose feet still touch the old-fashioned earth?

If you live in the city this is often a problem, and while a health food store can often provide you with a tasty (if expensive) solution, just as frequently it cannot. "Organic" egg production itself is often industrialized; the result—eggs that are undoubtedly healthier, but just as tasteless as the supermarket special. Try to find a store that deals with a specific farmer; or better still, take a drive and find the farmer yourself, or go to a local farmers' market. It is worth the effort. Though free-range and omega-3-enriched eggs (these eggs have come from chickens fed an omega-rich diet) have become increasingly available, the fact remains that they still do not rival a farm-fresh egg either in color or flavor.

A healthy egg not only tastes better but also is rich in protein, vitamins A, B, and D, and contains sodium, phosphorus, potassium, and lecithin—without contamination by cancerous cells and noxious chemicals. Fertile eggs are better for you than nonfertile eggs; but in mechanized egg production the rooster is just a nuisance—he eats too much and causes too much excitement among the lucky hens. And fertile eggs cannot be made to last for weeks and weeks the way nonfertile ones can—all in all a poor risk in our money-conscious society. If your child is allergic to nonfertile eggs, try searching out some fertile ones for him or her; often those who are allergic to one can tolerate the other.

Tell how fresh an egg is by putting it in a bowl of water. If it sinks, it is fresh. If it floats, it is rotten. If it wavers in the middle, it is okay—but cook it well, and eat it in a hurry!

Free-running chickens are also a tremendous natural insect control—one of the factors that makes their eggs and meat that much richer than the ersatz products of the egg-chicken factories of today.

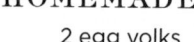 HOMEMADE MAYONNAISE

> 2 egg yolks
> 5 tablespoons vinegar or lemon juice
> 1 teaspoon salt
> 1 tablespoon curry powder
> 1½ cups olive oil, approximately

- Mix all ingredients except the olive oil in a blender, or preferably, with a hand mixer. Slowly add the olive oil as you beat the mixture, until the mayonnaise reaches the desired level of thickness—smooth and thick enough to work as a dipping sauce. As soon as you have reached the desired thickness (homemade mayonnaise will never be thick and gelatinous like conventional, store-bought mayonnaise), stop beating! Like whipping cream, mayonnaise can be taken too far and will separate from overbeating.
- Use as a sandwich spread, a dip for artichokes, or spread directly onto crackers for a delicious treat.

ELDERBERRY TEA   Although elderberry tea is the most generally used, the common elder (*Sambucus canadensis* and *S. nigra*) also offers up as tea its bark, roots, leaves, and flowers, all of which have curative powers. Indeed, so many different remedies have been ascribed to the elder that in England, for example, it was called "the medicine chest of the country people." An infusion of the bruised leaves is said to repel mosquitoes, gnats, and even mice. A brew made from the bark is a purgative and emetic. The berries, however, yield the most pleasing tea. They are high in vitamin C and can be used for the treatment of colds and influenza. They increase perspiration, are diuretic, and are therefore useful as a blood cleanser. Cooled elderberry tea is very soothing when applied to the eyes. The elder tree itself is steeped in legend. Old homes in England often have an elder planted nearby, for it was supposed to protect the inhabitants from witches. Judas is said to have hanged himself from an elder—the elder grows larger in Europe and the Middle East than in America—and the wood of the tree (there are several other sylvan candidates for the role) is reputed to have been used for the cross of Christ. Think on these things as you sip your cup of elderberry late at night by the fire.

EPAZOTE   Also known as the bean herb (due to its ability to reduce the gaseous effect of legumes), pigweed, or Mexican tea, epazote is a popular herb in both Mexico and the Caribbean. Epazote is pungent, with a strong flavor that some swear by and some consider to be an acquired taste. Use dried or fresh, in beans, quesadillas, sopes (fried cornmeal cakes), scrambled eggs, or fish dishes.

Medicinally, epazote can be taken as a tea to expel intestinal worms and to soothe digestion. It is said to be poisonous if ingested in extremely large quantities, but as the taste is so intensely pungent, the likelihood of an epazote overdose does not seem likely, so do not be afraid to flavor your cooking at will.

EUCALYPTUS TEA   The statuesque and aromatic eucalyptus tree, which sometimes reaches heights of 375 feet, is native to Australia and Tasmania. Now grown in many parts of the world, it is valued for its usefulness in reclaiming malarial areas and lands that are plagued by drought. And of course the eucalyptus has long had the distinction of its leaves being the sole diet of those wonderful koala bears. Though the long ovate leaves are reported to contain high amounts of hydrogen cyanide, their oil has long been recognized for its antiseptic qualities. The oil or crushed leaves can be applied to any surface skin wound with good results.

Tea made from the crushed leaves has an unusual bitter taste; it is said to be good for the digestion and useful for bronchial disorders. The vapors of the tea can also be inhaled in cases of asthma and chest congestion.

F

FAVA BEAN   Fava (or broad) beans have been cultivated in Europe since the Iron Age; they are now also grown in the United States. These large lima-shaped beans are usually sold dried and are a very rich source of vitamin B, protein, phosphorus, iron, and calcium. Excellent additions to soup, they can also be served alone—you may wish to cook them with a zestful sauce, however, for they tend to be bland in flavor.

Centuries ago Greeks and Romans believed that overindulgence in fava beans would impair the vision. Today among Mediterranean peoples (the most avid consumers of fava beans) there is a blood disorder known as favism, which is thought to be due to an overabundance of these beans in the diet. Such dire thoughts should not, however, interfere with enjoyment in moderation of this healthful and pleasant legume!

FAVA BEAN CASSEROLE

2 cups fava beans, dried

1 teaspoon salt

4 medium-size onions, sliced

4 tablespoons (½ stick) butter

½ teaspoon dried rosemary (or 1 teaspoon fresh, chopped)

½ teaspoon salt

⅛ teaspoon freshly ground black pepper

6 fresh tomatoes, peeled, seeded, and chopped (or 3 cups
        canned diced tomatoes with juice)

Soak beans overnight in water to cover. Put them in a pot with the salt and soaking water, add more water if necessary, and simmer covered for 2 hours or until tender. Meanwhile sauté the sliced onions in butter; add rosemary, salt, and pepper.

- When the fava beans are tender, mix them together with the onion mixture and the tomatoes. Turn into a casserole; cover and bake at 350 degrees for 1 hour for a hearty side vegetable dish or main course.
- Serves four to six.

FAVA BEAN
Pods, Seeds and Flowers approximately ⅔ size

FENNEL   Fennel can be found growing in almost every temperate climate; in California it grows wild in great profusion. Its uses are very similar to that of dill: the leaves are added to soups, salads, and fish. Toss a few fennel seeds in your next pot of baked beans—they will cut down on the gaseous effects of that dish. The seeds made into a tea to increase the milk supply in nursing mothers, have a sedative effect, aid digestion, and prevent infant colic.

Fennel tea is said to be particularly good for the eyes, either by using the tea as a compress or merely by drinking it regularly. Fennel tea also has a gentle laxative effect. To prepare, steep 1 teaspoon seeds in 1 cup of boiling water until desired strength is reached.

The licorice flavor of the fennel seed is particularly attractive to children; try giving your child branches of fennel (beware, the look-alike poison hemlock often grows nearby; you can tell hemlock by the large brown spots on its stem, said to be the blood of Aristotle, who was killed by being forced to drink hemlock tea) or a few seeds to chew on rather than the usual sugary licorice candy. Or chew it yourself—it sweetens the breath. A fennel branch placed under your next loaf of Italian bread as it bakes will impart a delicious subtle flavor.

FENNEL BREAD

1³/₄ cups lukewarm water

2 packages fresh yeast (or 2 tablespoons dry)

2¹/₄ teaspoons honey

2 tablespoons melted lukewarm butter

3¹/₂ cups unbleached white bread flour, sifted

1 teaspoon fennel seed

1¹/₂ teaspoons salt

Cornmeal

GLAZE:

1 egg yolk

2 teaspoons milk

4 teaspoons fennel seed

- Preheat oven to 350 degrees.
- Pour ¼ cup water over yeast and add ¼ teaspoon honey. Let it sit until the yeast begins to foam. Add 1½ cups lukewarm water, 2 teaspoons honey, and melted lukewarm butter. Stir in flour, fennel, and salt; mix well with a spoon or hands.

Turn out onto floured board and knead for about 10 minutes. Use more flour if necessary.

- Put into a large buttered bowl and cover with a towel. Let rise about 45 minutes or until double in bulk. Punch down and knead for 5 minutes. Shape into 2 round loaves. Place on a cookie sheet sprinkled with cornmeal. Cover and let rise for 30 minutes. Brush with glaze of egg yolk beaten with milk; sprinkle on 4 teaspoons fennel seed.
- Bake for 45 minutes or until brown.

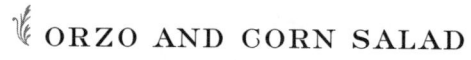 ## ORZO AND CORN SALAD

> 2 cloves garlic, chopped
> ½ cup chopped oil-packed sun-dried tomatoes, plus oil
> 1½ cups fresh corn
> 2 cups orzo, cooked
> 1 tablespoon fennel seeds, dry toasted
> Olive oil as needed
> Salt and pepper

- Sauté garlic in 2 tablespoons of sun-dried tomato oil, if available (otherwise, use olive oil). When garlic is tender, add corn and sauté for 2–3 minutes. Remove from heat. Cool. Add cooked orzo, tomatoes, and fennel seeds. Toss with either additional tomato oil or olive oil until grains are well coated. Salt and pepper to taste.
- Serves eight.

FENUGREEK SEED   Fruit of an herb native to the Mediterranean region, fenugreek seeds are most commonly used as tea for the relief of fever or to soothe irritated intestinal tracts. The tea can also be used as a gargle for sore throats. One teaspoon of seeds steeped in 2 cups boiling water will yield a delicate brew with a slightly licorice flavor. In India fenugreek seeds are used in curry sauces and the herb itself is eaten as a vegetable. The ground seeds can be mixed with water to a gelatinous paste and used as a poultice on wounds or inflamed areas of the skin. In the sixteenth century it was said that the aroma of the seeds kept away "noisome worms and creeping things."

FIG   The fig is a highly perishable fruit. Unless you live in a warm climate where figs flourish, you are likely to meet it most often in dried form. This wholesome practical food has been a staple for thousands of years. The Old Testament mentions it often and favorably, and it was a mainstay of the armies of the Roman Empire.

Figs are extremely rich in minerals. Their iron content makes them a good blood builder and useful in cases of anemia. Figs are also very effective as a laxative; but if your gastrointestinal tract is delicate, avoid this remedy, for the hundreds of tiny seeds in each fig are indigestible and can be irritating. Dried figs are an excellent candy substitute for children; best results are derived if you start giving figs as snacks at a very early age, before the child begins to have preconceived ideas about what a sweet should look and taste like. As with all dried fruit, careful tooth brushing is imperative, as the sugar tends to lodge between the teeth.

When purchasing dried figs, make certain that sulfur has not been used to speed up the drying and to preserve color and that the fig has not been dipped in sugar (to sweeten it) or water (to make it weigh more and seem moister). Properly dried figs have no need of these unhealthful methods.

FILBERT   The filbert and hazelnut belong to the same genus, and the distinctions between them are so minor that they can be used interchangeably. The filbert is said to ripen on August 22, which is St. Philbert's Day … from whence cometh the name of the nut. Filberts are small nuts with a smooth brown shell that yields easily to a nutcracker; there is no excuse for buying them preshelled! They are crisp, compact, and utterly delicious. Rich in protein and unsaturated oil, they pack such a lot of nutrition into a small space that they should be eaten in moderation. Add filberts to muesli cereal, cookies, and tortes.

FILBERT TORTE

4 eggs, separated
1 cup plus 2 tablespoons sugar (preferably raw sugar)
Zest of 1 lemon
3 cups ground filberts

- Preheat oven to 350 degrees. Oil and flour a 9-inch springform pan.
- Beat egg yolks until they are foamy. Pulverize the sugar in a blender, mix with lemon zest, then beat into the egg yolks until very light. Beat egg whites in a separate bowl until they are stiff but not dry. Stir 4 tablespoons of the beaten egg whites gently into egg yolk mixture.
- Fold the ground nuts (2 cups shelled filberts ground in a blender will yield the 3 cups ground nuts called for) into the egg whites, then fold the whites and

nuts into the egg yolks. Pour into the prepared pan. Bake for 40–50 minutes until golden. Cool before removing from pan.

꩜ Serves six.

FILÉ POWDER   Made from the powdered leaves of the sassafras tree, filé powder is an essential ingredient in Cajun cooking. The Choctaw Indians, native to Louisiana, were the original users of this bayou spice.

Reminiscent in taste to genuine root beer, filé powder acts as a thickener for soups, stews, and the traditional Cajun gumbo. It should be added after the dish has been removed from the heat, as the filè will turn tough and stringy when overcooked.

FISH   A good rule of thumb is, whenever pregnant women or children are advised to avoid something, it does not bode well for anyone! Enter the fish conundrum: so delicious, so healthy, so rich in protein and omega fatty acids, and yet, often so tainted by pollution. Excluding amalgam fillings and vaccinations, fish are a primary source of mercury exposure for humans. Mercury from industrial pollution is converted into methyl mercury in water and subsequently absorbed by the fish. According to the Environmental Protection Agency, the largest source of mercury pollution stems from coal-fired power plants; following closely behind are waste-incinerator plants. This is useful information to have, as it is not only ocean-dwelling fish that are contaminated, but freshwater fish as well. Fishermen should consider carefully the lengths of the rivers and water sources that they frequent and do thorough investigation before eating their catch. Large long-lived fish have the longest time to accumulate methyl mercury and are therefore the least safe. Shark, swordfish, king mackerel, albacore tuna, and freshwater bass and pike are among the worst offenders. Much safer are trap-caught shrimp, wild-caught salmon, yellowfin tuna, cod, and shellfish.

As with all food that we buy and then consume, it is important to be discerning about both the origins of the fish and the practices of the fishermen. For those of us who love to eat fish, the only option besides abstinence is to make a point of purchasing the right fish and then not to eat too much of it— a problem that is made somewhat easier by skyrocketing fish prices that reflect how many species of fish are dwindling. Chilean sea bass, for example, are rapidly disappearing. While many shellfish are best bought farmed—abalone, clams, mussels, and oysters, for example—some farm-raised fish are best avoided. Farm-raised salmon are a perfect example of a fish that should never be purchased. Fed antibiotics and additives to give their flesh the pink color we have come to expect, environmentally speaking, so far salmon farms have been a disaster. Escaped farm-raised salmon can push the local wild salmon out of their habitat. Wild salmon can also swim under the giant pens that contain the farm-raised salmon, becoming contaminated with deadly sea lice as they do so. The seabeds beneath the fisheries become polluted with fish waste. And let's face it, farm-raised salmon taste horrible when compared to the real thing.

Talk to your fish vendor and ask questions. How fresh are the fish? Where are they from? How are they being caught? Are they endangered? As time passes, so the laws and regulations change. Along with the increasing diminishment and contamination of fish from our seas and freshwater sources will come new laws to protect both the fish and the consumer. Keep abreast of these changes and make informed choices whether shopping at the fish market or fishing a local waterway.

APPLE-MARINATED SALMON FILLETS

6 (4–6 ounce) salmon fillets, 2–3 inches wide

2 cups apple juice

2 tablespoons Dijon mustard

¼ cup soy sauce

3 tablespoons fresh ginger, grated

1 tablespoon olive oil

1 tablespoon dried dill or thyme, or 2 tablespoons fresh

Marinate salmon fillets in the apple juice, mustard, soy, and ginger for 6–8 hours or overnight. Place salmon on baking sheet lined with parchment paper. Brush with olive oil. Sprinkle with dill or thyme. Bake salmon at 350 degrees for 8–10 minutes. Broil to color, 2–4 minutes.

Serves six.

CRAB CAKES

2 tablespoons butter

1 tablespoon oil

½ cup red bell pepper, seeded and chopped

½ cup yellow bell pepper, seeded and chopped

¼ cup chopped scallions

½ cup chopped parsley

1 cup fresh corn, cut from the cob

2 pounds crabmeat (pick clean of all shells)

2 tablespoons drained capers

4 tablespoons mustard

⅓–½ cup homemade or commercial mayonnaise

½ cup panko (these Japanese-style, coarse bread crumbs are available in Asian markets)

½ teaspoon salt

½ teaspoon pepper

- Melt butter and oil and sauté peppers and scallions until soft. Add corn kernels and cook for a few more minutes. Remove from stove and cool in a bowl.
- Mix crabmeat with capers, mustard, mayonnaise, parsley, salt, pepper, and panko. Combine with cooled vegetables. Add more panko if needed to bind. Cover and chill mixture for 30 minutes to 1 hour.
- Shape cooled mixture into cakes. (If you wish, you may dip cakes in a little panko before frying.) Depending on the size of the crab cakes, sauté in a combination of 4–8 tablespoons of butter and olive oil on both sides, cooking for about 10 minutes total. Drain and serve.
- Serves eight.

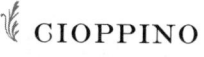 CIOPPINO

1 large onion, diced

3 cloves garlic, minced

1 medium green bell pepper, seeded and chopped

½ cup sliced celery

2 carrots, pared and sliced

5 tablespoons oil

2 pounds fresh tomatoes, peeled and seeded or 2 (1 pound) cans tomatoes

1 cup homemade tomato sauce (or one 8-ounce can tomato sauce)

1 tablespoon dried basil, crumbled

3 bay leaves

1 teaspoon salt

¼ teaspoon pepper

1 pound fish (any firm white fish)

1 dozen mussels

1 dozen clams

1½–2 cups dry white wine

1 pound shelled deveined shrimp

½ pound scallops

4 tablespoons fresh parsley, chopped

- In large pot, sauté onion, garlic, green pepper, celery, and carrots in oil until soft. Stir in tomatoes, tomato sauce, basil, bay leaves, salt, and pepper. Heat to boiling. Lower heat. Simmer 1 hour.
- While sauce simmers, remove skin (if any) from fish, and cut into bite-sized pieces. Scrub mussels and clams thoroughly. Stir wine into the sauce. Put mussels and clams on top. Steam for 5 or 10 minutes more until shells are fully opened. Throw out unopened clams and mussels. Add fish, shrimp, and scallops. Simmer for 10 minutes. Serve in bowls. Top with parsley.
- Serves six to eight.

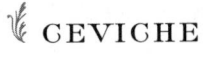

CEVICHE

¾ cup fresh lime juice

¼ cup olive oil

4 scallions, minced

2 tablespoons red onions, minced

1 red bell pepper, seeded and minced

4 tablespoons cilantro, chopped

1 pound bay scallops, whole or diced depending on preference

- Mix together all ingredients except scallops. When well mixed, add scallops. Marinate in the refrigerator for at least 4 hours.
- Drain. Serve on a chilled plate with sliced fresh tomatoes and arugula leaves. (May also be served in a hollowed-out tomato.)
- Serves four to six.

FLAXSEED   Flax has been cultivated since Stone Age times for the sake of its fibrous stems, which have long been used to make ropes and cloth. Until the eighteenth century, when cotton came to the forefront, flax was the most important vegetable fiber in the Western world. It is now grown primarily for use in the manufacture of luxury linen materials—and for its seeds and their oil.

The seeds of the flax plant are also known as linseed, and their oil is always called linseed oil. The brown shiny seeds were once used as a food item in the Middle East (where they were often eaten roasted), and we in this country are rediscovering their nutritional worth. High in unsaturated fatty acids, protein, phosphorus, niacin, and iron, flaxseeds are said to be particularly good for dry, brittle hair. Sprinkle the ground seeds on cereal, yogurt, or cottage cheese (they have a pleasant nutty flavor), and you may see your hair become thick and glossy in a matter of a few weeks. Flaxseeds are also good for constipation, as they swell and provide bulk for the intestines.

Flaxseeds can be bought whole and ground into meal in a blender, or purchased preground; the meal should always be refrigerated. Flaxseed oil, which abounds in omega-3 fatty acids, is the most potent way to reap the nutritional benefits of flax, and is said to be helpful for menopausal women, as well as providing all of the benefits mentioned for the flaxseed. As with the seed, just be sure to refrigerate, as flaxseed oil will quickly turn rancid.

Tea made from the seeds is said to be good for bronchial conditions and to have a laxative and soothing effect on the intestinal tract: Steep a tablespoon of flaxseeds in 2 cups boiling water for 15 minutes. Flaxseeds are very mucilaginous; a warm poultice made from the boiled seed or meal soothes sores, boils, and inflammations.

FLOUR   See individual flours, i.e., *Rye, Whole Wheat*, etc.

FO-TI   Fo-ti, also know as *he shou wu*, a member of the carrot family, is a low-lying herb that grows in the Eastern tropics. Proclaimed, like ginseng, to be a wondrous elixir, it is said to prolong life and vitality. One of its foremost exponents, Li Chung Yun, died in China in 1933 and was believed to have been 256 years old. Fo-ti is usually available in tablet form, and as a powder to be used as a tea.

FRUITS AND VEGETABLES, FRESH ORGANIC   The story of organic fresh fruits and vegetables, as available to us as buyers through commercial channels, is at the same time both hopeful and discouraging. On the one hand, more and more farmers are becoming aware of the long-term deleterious effects on their land of chemical fertilizers and pesticides and are swinging over to organic methods of farming; and these are not mere backyard gardeners but large-scale growers. This is great news for those of us who like our fruits and vegetables pure, fresh, and tasty, for it means that sky-high organic produce prices will gradually become lower and that there will be more things organic for everyone.

On the other hand, however, the picture is not so promising. As anyone who commonly buys organic produce is aware, the costs are easily twice as much as their nonorganic counterparts. While some would say this is a small price to pay for health and safety, the fact remains that for many of us buying everything organic is simply not an option. Not everyone can afford to spend upwards of ten dollars for one melon, or three dollars for a single artichoke. What to do about it? First, try to buy fruits and vegetables that are in season in the area where you live. They are more likely to be fresh-picked, and the prices of in-season produce are consistently lower than when trying to buy out of season. Also, the sources will probably be nearby, and you can visit them and satisfy yourself as to their integrity and quality. Of course, there are many items that we have grown accustomed to eating that can never be local—bananas, or citrus fruit, or avocados if you live in New York. In this case, it is even more important to purchase these items organically grown only, as many imported fruits and vegetables are contaminated with pesticides that are now outlawed in the United States that are known to cause cancer and nerve damage, both in those who ingest the pesticides and in the farmworkers who have to handle them.

One might well wonder whether in the end it is worth all the time and money to buy organic fruits and vegetables. Often the flavor of a well-grown tomato or orange is so superlative that it seems worth any amount of trouble and money to obtain it. Other times, however, you will find yourself with an organically raised bunch of spinach or celery that frankly just does not taste that much different from its chemically raised counterpart. And then the natural reaction is to quickly beat it back to the supermarket and its easier prices. En route, however, remember that you will then be feeding yourself and your family any one of some forty-two chemicals that the United States Department of Agriculture has deemed "safe" to a certain level of tolerance. Often this level is passed, but only occasionally are foods officially detected and recalled. Conventional produce is also likely to be gassed to hasten "ripening," to be dyed, soaked in antibiotic fluids to delay ripening, packed in wrappings treated with toxic materials to prevent rotting—in addition to all the pesticides that cannot be washed or peeled off, for they penetrate through the roots to the very heart of the matter.

Add to the risk of pesticide-laden fruits and vegetables the now hotly debated rise in GMO, or genetically modified organisms, foods to the marketplace, and we have a new reason to go rushing toward organically grown and non-GMO produce. Though it is true that gardeners, farmers, and scientists have been creating "hybrid" plants for generations—crossing broccoli with cauliflower, for instance—this is not at all the same as crossing a gene from a totally unrelated species with the genetic material of another. Want some concrete examples of GMOs that are grown right here in the United States? Spider genes in goats. Fish genes in tomatoes. Rat and human genes in trout. Mouse and human genes in potatoes. So far, thirty countries have banned, or propose to ban GMO crops. Let us hope that the United States has the willpower and the wisdom to do the same. In the meantime, be sure to buy organic and GMO-free corn, potato, and soy products, as these are increasingly grown from genetically modified seeds.

A last note on organically raised fresh produce: Take the occasional wormhole as evidence of a healthful upbringing. Do not demand chemically induced perfect appearance in organic fruits and vegetables; but do always insist on freshness. And remember, by buying organically grown, GMO-free produce, you are not only protecting your own health and the health of your family, but you are protecting the farmworkers, the people who live near the farms, the earth's water supplies, and the very soil beneath your feet.

G

GARLIC Garlic is a bulbous plant related to the onion; it has a strong (and to the garlic enthusiast, irresistible) odor and flavor. Miraculous healing and health-giving powers have been attributed to garlic since Babylonian times. The wandering Israelites mourned the cherished garlic they had left behind in Egypt. It was a mainstay in the diet of the builders of the pyramids, and of ancient Greek and Roman soldiers and sailors—no Phoenician would set sail without a healthy store of garlic on board. In medieval times garlic was burned to disinfect houses visited by the plague and to ward off sickness in general.

Garlic is useful in the relief of bronchial coughs, asthma, and head colds; prepare a syrup of garlic juice, made from pressed garlic that has been filtered through a cheesecloth, and honey and take as needed. For braver types, garlic can be eaten raw; for the more reticent sufferer, garlic pills are available in health food stores. Garlic is an excellent stimulant to digestion and has an antiseptic action on the intestines. Its antiseptic qualities are also useful externally; poultices made of crushed garlic are recommended for everything from smallpox and whooping cough to poison ivy and pimples. In World War II the British are said to have successfully used quantities of fresh garlic to prevent infection and hasten healing of soldiers' wounds. However, avoid applying fresh garlic directly to the skin, as it may cause irritation. Garlic is recognized as a laxative and is said to prevent intestinal gas.

If you like to chew garlic—this is reputed to give the most beneficial results—follow it down with some parsley or mint or fennel seeds if you respect the noses of those around you. Garlic can be used for cooking in a myriad of manners: Chop it, crush it, squeeze it, use it whole, or merely rub it. Squeezing it through a garlic press gives the most pungent result, so restrict the amount you use accordingly. For the subtlest effect rub the cut end of the clove on bread, meat, the salad bowl.

GINGER   Ginger has long been cultivated in tropical Asia. Marco Polo reported it growing in China, and Europeans raced over the "spice routes" to obtain this aromatic delicacy. It is now most commonly grown in Jamaica, Africa, South America, and the West Indies. Its shallow-growing rhizome is the valued part, which we know as the ginger root. The tea, made from fresh or dried diced root of ginger, is a good tonic for digestion, delayed menstruation, nerves, and nausea. Sweetened with honey and with a slice of lemon added, it is a spicy pleasant brew. Add a few bits of ginger to a pot of chamomile tea for a real treat. Small pieces of ginger may be chewed as an aid to digestion and to alleviate motion sickness—these are hot on the tongue, but strangely delicious.

Try adding ½ teaspoon of thin-sliced ginger root to butter before pouring in the eggs for scrambling, or add a teaspoonful to your rice as it cooks for a delicate mysterious flavor. Powdered ginger is used most often in curries and cookies—and of course in gingerbread and gingersnaps.

Why not make your own ginger ale? Without harmful sugars and preservatives, you will have this delicious drink as it once was and should be.

GINGER ALE

> Rind and juice of 4 lemons
> 2 quarts water
> 1 cup chopped fresh ginger, unpeeled (or reconstituted from
>   dried root)
> 6 tablespoons honey
> Mint

- Cut lemon rind in paper-thin strips. Pour boiling water over the chopped ginger and lemon rind; steep for 5 minutes. Strain and stir in the honey. Chill. Add lemon juice, ice, and sprigs of mint.
- Serves eight.
- *Note:* For carbonated ginger ale, steep ginger and lemon peel in only 1 quart boiling water. When serving, add 1 quart cold soda water.

GINGER ROOT
life size

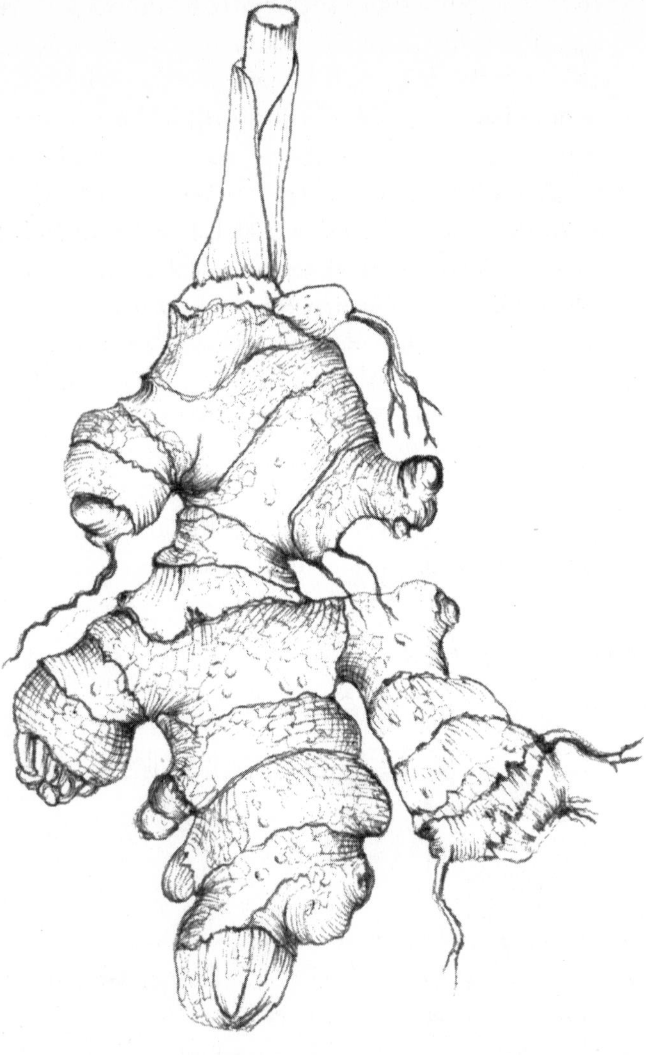

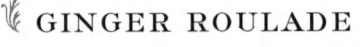

GINGER ROULADE

- 1 sheet mountain shepherd bread (lavash), available in health food stores and some supermarkets
- 1 (8-ounce) package cream cheese, whipped in Cuisinart or blender for 15–30 seconds
- 1 bunch watercress, large stems removed, washed, and spun very dry
- 1 (6-ounce) jar pickled ginger, with all liquid squeezed out

- On the sheet of lavash, spread cream cheese in a square. Do not spread cheese to the edges—leave 1–2 inches clear on each edge. Place watercress one piece at a time in a single layer on top of cream cheese. Then place pickled ginger on top of watercress in a single layer.
- Trim the edge nearest to you and begin to roll the bread as tightly as possible, being careful not to break the bread. (If you do—not to worry—just keep on going. It will stick back together.) Roll half of the bread and cut that roll off. Continue to roll the remainder of the bread. Trim far end when roll is finished, then trim both ends of each roll. Cut each roll in half.
- Slice into ½–¾-inch rounds. Lovely as an hors d'oeuvre.

DELICIOUS CRUDITÉ DIP

1 inch fresh ginger, grated
¼ cup cilantro, chopped
2 tablespoons sesame oil
2 tablespoons sweet rice vinegar
1 cup homemade mayonnaise (see recipe in book)

- Mix all ingredients together at least 4 hours before using. Chill. Serve with cut up colorful vegetables. Also delicious with chilled poached shrimp.

GINKGO BILOBA   A common addition to Japanese temple gardens, the ginkgo biloba is considered to be one of the world's oldest species of tree, and can be traced back to the time of dinosaurs. Ginkgo-leaf extract is best known for its usefulness in the treatment of memory loss and has been used to treat Alzheimer's disease, age-related dementia, as well as the short-term memory loss common to many. Ginkgo is also used in the treatment of PMS, vertigo, and high cholesterol. Ginkgo is available in pill, capsule, and tincture form. The fresh ginkgo nut is also edible and has a mild, slightly sweet flavor that is widely enjoyed in both Japanese and Chinese cuisine.

GINSENG   Miraculous curative powers are attributed to the ginseng plant, which has held a leading position in Chinese herbal medicine for over fifty centuries. The root of the plant is the most valued part (although the leaves and flowers can be used for tea that echoes the qualities of the root, in milder form). The root is gnarled and strangely shaped, and the more it resembles the shape of a man, the more valuable it is considered. Perfect roots of this type sell for thousands of dollars on the ever-fluctuating ginseng market. Ginseng was discovered growing wild in America in the eighteenth century. Although American ginseng is considered to be inferior in quality to the Asiatic, when one considers the high prices of Asiatic ginseng, the American plant begins to look pretty good! The root has been brought under cultivation on both sides of the earth, but the cultivated root is considered inferior to the wild root.

Ginseng is reputed to ease childbirth pains, relieve menopausal symptoms, and increase sexual desire. It is also used as a disease preventative, to aid digestion and strengthen the stomach, to promote appetite, to ward off constipation— and as a general tonic for just about any complaint in men, women, and children.

Ginseng is sold in liquid, powder, capsule, and root forms. The liquid and powder may be dissolved and taken as tea or mixed with other beverages. The root may be chewed or chopped and boiled for use as a tea.

GLUTEN FLOUR   Gluten flour is wheat flour with the starch removed. It is used for bread making by those who wish to restrict their carbohydrate intake. It can also be used to make gluten dishes, which are high in protein and therefore useful in vegetarian diets.

Gluten is an elastic protein substance that is present in all wheat flours to a greater or lesser degree. Spring or hard wheat is high in gluten, and this is what makes it a good flour for making bread; the gluten surrounds the bubbles of fermenting yeast and yields light airy loaves. Winter wheat or all-purpose flour is rather low in gluten and therefore does not lend itself to bread making, for the loaves would be crumbling and heavy. Gluten flour comes in handy when using flours that are low in gluten, such as corn, soy, rye, oat, and barley; for each cup of low-gluten flour, add ½ cup gluten flour in exchange for an equal amount of wheat flour, and your loaves will avoid the heaviness that these low-gluten flours tend to produce.

To make gluten for vegetarian dishes, mix gluten flour or wheat flour with water to create a stiff dough; soak and knead in cold running water until the water is clear of starch and all that is left is a glutinous ball of dough. Of course, this is a quicker process with gluten flour than with wheat flour. The dough is sliced and steamed or parboiled, then treated like a slice of meat to be sautéed or ground and shaped into patties or loaves.

Although gluten has the advantages of being high in protein and low in carbohydrates, it is also low in minerals—they are lost during the soaking process of extracting the gluten from the wheat flour.

GLUTEN-SOY BREAD

1 tablespoon dried yeast (or 1 compressed yeast cake)

1½ cups lukewarm water

1 tablespoon honey

1 tablespoon pressed vegetable oil

1 teaspoon salt

1½ cups gluten flour

¾ cup soy flour

¾ cup whole wheat flour

- Preheat oven to 350 degrees.
- Dissolve yeast in warm water and let it rest until it begins to foam. Stir in honey and oil. Sift in salt, gluten flour, and soy flour and stir very thoroughly.
- Spread the whole wheat flour on a kneading board. Put batter on board, flour your hands, and knead for about 8 minutes, adding more whole wheat flour if necessary. The more you knead, the lighter the bread will be.
- Place it to rise in a covered oiled bowl, in a warm spot, until double in bulk. This will take an hour to an hour and a half. Then punch down the dough, form it into a loaf, and place it in an oiled bread pan. Let it rise again until the dough is just a little higher than the top of the pan. Bake for about 50 minutes.
- This high-protein, low-starch loaf is so light and tasty—no one would ever suspect it of being a "health" bread!
- Makes one loaf.

GOAT MILK   Goat milk, as well as the cheeses made from it, are easier for the human body to assimilate than cow milk. Nearer in composition to mother's milk, it can often be tolerated by infants when cow milk is rejected. Goat husbandry has not become so industrialized as that of cows; therefore, chances are that the goats will be healthier and produce milk of higher quality.

Aside from their outstanding health value, goat milk, cheese, and yogurt can have a particularly "earthy" taste that many people covet (and others abhor).

GOLDENROD TEA   When used externally, this tea has a long-standing reputation for its healing power on wounds. When taken internally, it has been successful with problems of the kidneys and ulcers as well as easing cases of hay fever. *Solidago odura* and *S. virgaurea* are the species of goldenrod most commonly used. One teaspoon dried flower tops should be boiled for

1 minute, steeped for 15, then strained and served. The tea has a sweet, pleasant flavor.

Goldenrod tea is sometimes also known as solidago tea, after the generic name for goldenrod. This herb is best avoided by those suffering from kidney disorders.

GOLDENSEAL   The medicinal properties of this wild North American plant (*Hydrastis canadensis*) lie in its bright yellow roots. It is considered to be one of our most valuable and versatile herbs. The Cherokee Indians brought it to the attention of the invading Europeans; Native Americans had long valued it as a golden dye and as a veritable cure-all. Goldenseal is antiseptic and can be applied externally to wounds, eczema, the healing belly button of a newborn infant, and poison oak and ivy. It can also be used as an eye bath, a douche, or a gargle. Its laxative properties make it a good bowel conditioner. It is also soothing to ulcers of the stomach and intestines. Applied to the gums, it will ease inflammation—but your mouth will turn bright yellow, so beware!

There is no concealing the fact that goldenseal (it is sold in powder form or tincture) is extremely bitter in taste. Mix 1 to 3 teaspoons in water or orange juice, take a brave breath, and gulp it down. Best consult an herbalist for the dosage appropriate to your specific needs, for goldenseal is a true medicine and not to be toyed with. Do not take goldenseal when pregnant, and do not take for more than two weeks at a time, as goldenseal has been shown to have antibiotic properties that can diminish healthy intestinal flora after prolonged use. Goldenseal is a very potent healing herb, and small doses are recommended.

GOMASIO   The macrobiotic manner of eating emphasizes the need for salt in the diet but at the same time calls for limited intake of liquid. It is said that when salt is taken in the form of gomasio—a mixture of sea salt and sesame seeds—thirst is prevented. You do not have to be macrobiotic to enjoy this delicious seasoning. It is available preprepared in health food stores. Or make your own—fresh and superb.

GOMASIO

⅛ cup sea salt

1 cup raw sesame seeds, unhulled

Grind salt into a powder with a mortar and pestle (the Japanese use a special ridged ceramic bowl, a *suribachi*, for this). Toast the salt in a heavy frying pan until it shines; remove to another container.

◆ Roast sesame seeds in frying pan until they are lightly toasted; stir constantly with a wooden spoon to prevent burning. Grind seeds coarsely in mortar or *suribachi*; add salt and continue grinding until most—but not all—of the seeds are pulverized. The idea is for each grain of salt to be coated with sesame oil.

◆ Store in refrigerator or cool place. Use whenever salt is called for.

GRAHAM FLOUR   Graham flour is a whole wheat flour made from winter wheat. Similar to whole wheat pastry flour in the fineness of its grind, it usually contains more bran. The size of the bran granules will vary from mill to mill (the making of graham flour remains an individualized process in an age of standardization!). If a recipe calls for graham flour and there is none in the cupboard, whole wheat pastry flour can be substituted, cup for cup.

The flour was named after Sylvester Graham, an American physician who in the early nineteenth century was already fighting for dietary reform. He chaffed against the horrors of useless white bread: Thousands of people, he said, "eat the most miserable trash that can be imagined, in the form of bread, and never seem to think that they can possibly have anything better, nor even that it is an evil to eat such vile stuff as they do." And much of our bread has certainly gone downhill even from the "vileness" of Graham's day! Graham also lent his name to the graham cracker, once a most nutritious item, now gone the way of all devitalized bakery products. Why not try stepping back in time to make your own?

❦ GRAHAM CRACKERS

    8 tablespoons (1 stick) butter
    $2/3$ cup "raw" or brown sugar, firmly packed
    2 cups graham flour
    $1/2$ teaspoon salt
    $1/2$ teaspoon baking powder
    $1/4$ teaspoon ground cinnamon
    $1/2$ cup water

◆ Cream butter and sugar well. Sift together dry ingredients and add to creamed mixture, alternating with the water. Mix well. Let stand for 30 minutes.

◆ Preheat oven to 350 degrees. Oil a cookie sheet.

◆ Roll out dough on floured board to ⅛-inch thickness. Cut in squares or rounds, and bake for about 20 minutes, or until lightly browned.

◆ Makes about three dozen.

GROUND IVY TEA   A favorite remedy in times gone by, this bitter brew has been recommended for a variety of ailments—coughs, blood and kidney disorders, rheumatism, sciatica, gout, indigestion. The herbalist Nicholas Culpeper proclaimed it "a singular herb for all inward wounds" and assured that it would expel "melancholy by opening the stoppings of the spleen."

The tonic effects of this tea may be explained by its very high mineral content. It is also rich in vitamin C and was once used by painters to prevent lead poisoning; it is now known that vitamin C combines with lead and enables it to be excreted from the body.

Because of its bitter taste, ground ivy is usually mixed with other herb teas, such as sage, rosemary, or chamomile. Or mix it cold with orange juice. Taken cold it is an excellent bitters to stimulate the appetite.

At one time used in the processing of beer, ground ivy (*Glechoma hederacea*) is also known as gill-over-the-ground, alehoof, or gill (from the French *guiller*, to ferment beer).

GUARANA   Reputed to improve concentration, act as a painkiller, and relieve the discomfort of heat, guarana provides a long-lasting energy boost that is said to be superior to the rapid highs and lows provided by caffeine. Guarana contains guaranine—a chemical stimulant similar to caffeine. It offers instant stimulation and can keep you awake for hours. But it has similar side effects as caffeine, and an overdose can be dangerous to the health. Popular in Brazilian soft drinks, guarana comes from South America in a powder that looks like chocolate and is mixed with other drinks to mask its bitter taste. Guarana nutritional supplements are best avoided if one is suffering from heart disease or high blood pressure.

H

HAWTHORN BERRY TEA There are many different types of hawthorn bushes and trees throughout the temperate zones of the earth. They bear berries (or haws) that are usually red and rarely eaten by humans—though they are popular with wildlife. Some types make good jam. Hawthorn berry tea is high in vitamin C and therefore good for colds. It has also been used to alleviate heart conditions, improve circulation, and lower high blood pressure (the bark, too, is sometimes used).

The thorny hawthorn is said to have made up the crown of Christ. French peasants used to claim they could hear the hawthorn tree moan and cry on Good Fridays.

HAZELNUT See *Filbert.*

HERBS The leaves, seeds, or flowers of various aromatic plants are known as herbs; they make cooking an exciting adventure. Herbs can enhance or destroy a recipe. Too heavy a hand will smother all other flavors; too light a touch will leave you with boring blandness. A pinch of a dried herb will go a long way; use about one-third as much of a dried herb as you would of a fresh one.

Fresh herbs are of course always to be preferred over dried ones, for in the drying process essential flavors are always lost to some extent. When buying dried herbs, try to find a small, conscientious herb farm where herbs are treated gently and with care. Commercially dried herbs are crushed and dried on hot steel cylinders, and the heat destroys essential flavor-producing oils. Herbs distributed by large commercial concerns are also likely to have been sitting on a store shelf for untold lengths of time. Dried herbs should be used within eight months of drying, then refreshed with newly dried ones. Always store in airtight containers in a cool place; over the stove—a most handy spot—is unfortunately a bad place, because the herbs get too hot.

When using herbs in cooking or in teas, remember that the strength of an herb varies greatly depending on where it is grown, when it is picked, and how it is dried. See also individual herbs.

HIBISCUS TEA   See *Karkade Tea.*

HIZIKI   Also known as hijiki, this black, stringlike seaweed, sometimes known as black rice, is served as a vegetable. Hiziki is iodine and mineral rich and can be reconstituted in water and added to soups, salads, and stir-fries.

🌿 PAN-SIMMERED HIZIKI
  2 cups hiziki
  2 tablespoons sesame oil

- Soak hiziki in cold water for 15 minutes, then cut into bite-size pieces, and sauté in sesame oil, on medium heat for five minutes. Let the pan cool down, add the soaking water, and simmer on low for about 1 hour.
- Serve alone with tamari sauce or add to any other sautéed vegetable.
- Serves four.

HONEY   After centuries of being upstaged by refined cane sugar, honey is once again coming into its own. The Greeks regarded it as food fit for gods, and men who consumed it became just a little bit godlike. Well, physiologically at any rate, we are finding that the Greeks were not far wrong. Honey is *good* for your body, and who knows, maybe for your spirit as well. Certainly there is something very comforting about a big pot full of thick amber honey sitting in the middle of a table.

Here are some of the healthful attributes of honey. It is easy on the digestive organs, for the bees have already digested it for you. It is antiseptic and gives relief to burns and skin abrasions and bee stings (yes!). As a gargle, it soothes sore throats. It is a gentle laxative. It contains many minerals, such as copper, iron, manganese, silica, chlorine, calcium, sodium, potassium, phosphorus, magnesium—dark honey is said to have a higher mineral content than light honey. Honey that has not been filtered contains vitamin C from its pollen. Chewing of the honeycomb is beneficial to sinus and hay fever congestion.

The surest way to get pure untreated, unheated honey is to buy it in the comb. Next best, try to get honey that is unfiltered (it will still be cloudy with healthful pollen) and unheated (the minerals will remain intact). Bees do not have a high resistance to insecticides; when exposed they usually die rather than carry the poison back to the hive—hard on the poor bees, but fortunate for the human beings. As can be expected these days, however, many unhealthful practices have invaded the business of beekeeping. Honey is often subjected to high heat to prevent it from granulating (if your honey granulates, that means it is alive and well and you only have to put it in a pot of warm water for it to liquefy again)—to all effects, it is killed. Instead of brushing the bees off the comb to extract the honey from the hive, poisons are often used to make the bees leave. Then the bees, if they live through this treatment, become weak and disease-prone and are treated with sulfur and antibiotics, which are passed on to the honey. So be careful where you buy your honey. Buy from a health food store dealing with a small apiary that handles its honey ethically and with respect for this godlike substance.

Cooking with honey is unfortunately quite a problem. There are many recipes that just do not work with honey. Cookies won't be as crunchy, nor cakes as light, nor will preserves jell as firmly. How to get honey into your diet and sugar out? First use it in tea and coffee and on cereal and toast. Then start introducing it into your cooking. Bread accepts honey nicely; substitute it for the white sugar called for. When using honey in desserts, avoid types such as buckwheat and heather that have strong flavors—the milder, the better, so that the honey will remain merely a sweetener and not submerge the taste of the dessert. A general rule of thumb is to substitute three-quarters of the amount of sugar called for with honey (i.e., in a recipe calling for 1 cup of sugar, use ¾ cup honey and eliminate the sugar), and cut down the liquid in the recipe by one-fifth. If you are doubtful about going all the way with honey in a certain batch of cookies, try using half sugar and half honey—you'll have the best of both worlds. Remember that every time you think of a way to use honey instead of sugar you have done your body a big favor. A note of caution! Honey cannot be digested by children under twelve months of age and can cause infant botulism. Never, under any circumstances, feed honey to infants.

HONEY-YEAST ROLLS

1 package fresh yeast (or 1 tablespoon dry)

¼ cup warm water

1 cup milk

4 tablespoons (½ stick) butter

⅓ cup honey

1 teaspoon salt

2½ cups whole wheat flour, sifted

2½ cups unbleached white flour, sifted

2 eggs, well beaten

Dissolve yeast in warm water. Scald milk in a small saucepan and add butter and honey. Let butter melt. Cool milk mixture to lukewarm temperature and add to yeast and water; add salt and 3 cups of combined flour. Mix well and add beaten eggs. Add rest of flour. Mix well with spoon or hands for 5 minutes. Knead until satin smooth. Place in buttered bowl; cover and let rise for about 50 minutes or until double in bulk.

Punch down dough and form into round balls about the size of a golf ball. Place separately on a buttered cookie sheet or close together in a round pan that has been buttered. Cover and let rise again for about 30 minutes. Bake at 375 degrees for 20 minutes or until nicely browned.

Delicious served hot or rewarmed, for dinner or breakfast. These freeze well, too.

Makes about 32 rolls.

ACORN SQUASH WITH HONEY

2 medium acorn squash

4 tablespoons honey

4 teaspoons butter

4 teaspoons sherry (or dry vermouth)

Salt and pepper

Preheat oven to 400 degrees. Cut each squash in half, remove seeds, and place the 4 halves cut side up in a baking dish filled with ½ inch water.

Put 1 tablespoon honey, 1 teaspoon butter, and 1 teaspoon sherry in the center of each piece. Sprinkle with salt and freshly ground pepper; bake for 40 minutes or until tender when pricked with a fork.

Serves four.

CRANBERRY SAUCE

4 cups fresh cranberries

$3/4$ cup honey

1 teaspoon ground cinnamon

$1/2$ teaspoon ground nutmeg

$1/8$ teaspoon ground allspice

Juice and chopped pulp of 2 medium oranges

$1/2$ teaspoon lemon juice

Mix all ingredients in a saucepan and cook covered until the cranberries are very tender—about 45 minutes. Serve well chilled.

Makes about 3 cups.

HOPS TEA   Although hops may be best known as an ingredient of beer, if you are feeling nervous and sleepless, then perhaps what you need is a hot cup of hops tea, and then to sleep on a hops pillow. Hops is a perennial vine that came by way of China to Europe and America. Its conelike fruit is used for beer making; or chopped, as a nervine tea—or as a pillow stuffing! Such pillows gained popularity after George III of England announced that cares of state vanished with a sound night's sleep on a mound of hops.

The tea, which is quite bitter, is above all esteemed for its sedative and tranquilizing properties. It is also useful in cases of indigestion, neuralgia, and liver ailments. Purportedly it will also help to subdue sexual desire, should that be one of your problems. The tea can be used as a poultice to ease external inflammations, as well. To brew hops tea, steep 1 teaspoon hops in 1 cup boiling water for about 15 minutes.

HOREHOUND TEA   The leaves of this herb of the mint family are covered with a white hoary felt—hence its popular name, horehound. The bitter, spicy leaves have long been used as a remedy for colds, coughs, and asthmatic conditions. Strong infusions of this herbal tea are diuretic and laxative—so if it's a cold you have, don't make the tea *too* strong. For coughs—both child and adult—steep a tablespoon of crushed horehound leaves in 2 cups boiling water for 20 minutes; add honey and take as needed.

Horehound candy is good for scratchy throats. Make certain, however, to purchase it sweetened with honey rather than sugar.

HORSERADISH   The root of this perennial herb may cause your tongue to burn and your eyes to sting—but what a delicious taste! Horseradish originated in Eastern Europe, but it is now grown and eaten in almost all parts of the world. Grated and mixed with vinegar and salt, it is the traditional accompaniment for boiled meats, and corned beef. Added to cream sauces and mayonnaise, it is a fitting partner to all sorts of fish dishes. When buying prepared horseradish, be careful that it is without noxious additives; study the labels.

Horseradish is extremely rich in vitamin C and also contains a large amount of potassium. It is diuretic, stimulates the appetite, and aids digestion. Its high content of mustard oil makes it a potential irritant to the digestive organs; if yours are weak, go easy with this herb. It will help to dissolve phlegm in the throat: Mix 1 teaspoon horseradish with 1 teaspoon lemon juice and take a couple of times a day. Horseradish mixed with vinegar was once used to make freckles fade away.

HUCKLEBERRY TEA   The huckleberry bush is hardly distinguishable from its botanical relative, the blueberry, and the medicinal values of the two teas are identical. In ancient times both the berries and the leaves were infused; now only the leaves are used to make a tea that is an astringent in cases of diarrhea and is said to be useful in the treatment of diabetes because of its insulin content. To brew tea, steep 1 teaspoon leaves in 2 cups boiling water for 20 minutes.

IRISH MOSS   Irish moss, also known as carrageen, is a seaweed that is very high in calcium and iodine. It is most commonly used as a thickening agent, in the same manner as agar-agar, flour, or arrowroot starch. Carrageen is one of the few emulsifying agents found in industrialized foods that are beneficial to health. Powdered Irish moss is traditionally used to make the famous blanc-mange and is a useful jelling agent in other custards and puddings. While blanc-mange may not be as popular or well known as it once was, it is a dish worth experimenting with for those who like to try new things in the kitchen and are drawn to timeworn culinary delights.

Irish moss tea is made by steeping the dried moss in boiling water; strain and add honey for a brew that is helpful in cases of diarrhea and for kidney and bladder problems.

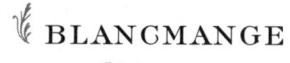 **BLANCMANGE**

³⁄₄ cup Irish moss
4 cups milk
Dash of salt
½ teaspoon lemon or pure vanilla extract
Honey and cream or fruit

- Soak moss in cold water 5 minutes. Drain and tie moss in cheesecloth. Put in top part of double boiler with the milk and salt. Put over boiling water and cook, covered, 30 minutes.
- Remove bag and discard. Add flavoring to milk mixture, pour into bowl and chill until firm.
- Serve with honey and cream.
- Makes four servings.

J

JUICE, FRUIT AND VEGETABLE   Fruit and vegetable juices provide valuable nutrients in an easily assimilated form. The only trouble is, through processing and storage their health value is severely impaired. Commercial juices are usually made from the frozen concentrate of insecticide-sprayed fruits and vegetables, preservatives, artificial coloring, and water (usually *lots* of it). Juices labeled as "all-natural" are often a put-on, for many of them are not made from fresh produce but from concentrate; and they have to undergo heating, which destroys nutrients (any fresh juice will start to ferment unless it is treated by heating and/or preservatives). Whenever possible purchase organic juice, whether fresh, bottled, or frozen concentrate.

The best way to obtain full benefit from your juice is to invest in a juicer and make your own. A juicer is an expensive item, but well worth it to those who become aware of the joys of fresh juice. Then any combination of fruits and vegetables that hits your fancy or your nutritional needs can be made on the spot. Try mixing apple, carrot, and celery; watercress, cabbage, and celery; cucumber, lettuce, and carrot; apple and potato (all the starch remains in the pulp and its juice is rich in vitamin C); add bean sprouts to any concoction for vitamin C and minerals. Fresh juices should be enjoyed immediately upon making, for they quickly lose nutrients, even under refrigeration.

JUNIPER BERRY   The bluish-gray berry—fresh or dried—of the juniper evergreen tree (*Juniperis communis*) may be used for making a tea that is said to be good for kidney and bladder trouble. Used as a spray, juniper tea is said to fumigate sick rooms; and as a gargle, to prevent catching a disease to which you have been exposed. To prepare the tea steep 1 teaspoon berries in 1 cup boiling water for 2–4 minutes. Strain and serve.

The juniper berry is also a gourmet cooking item. Its flavor is strong and pungent, and a few berries will carry you a long way. Juniper berries complement most meat dishes and are used in stuffings for everything from Cornish game hen to goose. A half-dozen berries dropped into your rice pot will make a flavorful accompaniment to a dinner of game. They are also used in meat marinades—if soaked too long, they begin to have a strong resemblance to their most famous offspring, gin.

K

KAMUT   According to legend, a United States airman, soon after the end of World War II, discovered kamut grains in an Egyptian tomb, mailed the kernels to a friend, who subsequently passed them on to his father, who just so happened to be a Montana farmer. The farmer planted the kernels, harvested the wheat, and kamut was born again.

Because of governmental policies and the realities of survival, farmers around this same time period were actively switching over to high-yield hybridized wheat, a trend that virtually eliminated ancient grains from the market. And yet, despite these trends, kamut (some sixty years later) has managed to reassert itself into the field and the cupboard.

Two to three times the size of common wheat, kamut is higher in protein, amino acids, vitamins, and minerals, and is reportedly easier to digest than common wheat. Because kamut is naturally sweet, less sugar is needed when it is used in cereals, breads, and other baked goods, as there is no need to mask the bitter flavor that is common to most other wheat products. While the tale of kernels discovered in a tomb may not be true, the fact remains that nutritionally speaking, kamut is truly a grain befitting of kings.

KARKADE TEA   A favorite drink from North Africa made from a type of hibiscus, this brilliant red drink has a flavor that is similar to lemon and is delicious served hot or cold. Use 1 teaspoonful tea to 1 cup briskly boiling water and steep for only a few minutes. Strain and serve in glasses so that you can enjoy the rich color. Karkade combines very well with rose hips; try mixing the two for a delicious tea.

KASHA   See *Buckwheat*.

KEFIR   Kefir is a delicious fermented milk. It is similar in taste to yogurt, and some people consider it more nutritious. It is certainly easier to make, for the milk does not have to be heated and the temperature does not have to be controlled. Kefir grains are available in health food stores, with instructions for making kefir at home.

Kefir has long been used in Eastern Europe, the Middle East, and parts of Asia. Persian women drank kefir to keep their complexions fresh and clear. It is said to be useful for inflammatory conditions of the stomach, intestinal tract, and liver. In the same way as yogurt, its friendly bacteria do away with unfriendly bacteria in the intestines. Kefir is helpful in curing both constipation and diarrhea; fresh kefir should be taken for constipation and kefir more than four days old will prove helpful with diarrhea.

KELP   Kelp is a brown seaweed that is available in dried, powdered, or tablet form. It contains an enormous number of minerals that are extremely important to our bodies. The best known is iodine, followed by chlorine, copper, zinc, potassium, iron, sodium, magnesium, manganese, and others. The better the seawater (a sorry problem today), the better the kelp. A great deal of kelp is eaten in Japan, where thyroid or goiter problems are rare due to the high intake of iodine in the seaweed. Kelp is often prescribed for weight loss, as it is said to reduce fat without harm to the body. It must be noted, however, that this takes place over a long period of time and instant results should not be expected.

Granular or powdered kelp may be added to bread or any baked goods (half a teaspoon to a cup of flour—and eliminate the salt—is a good start). It can also be sprinkled on cheese, salad, soup, vegetables, or added to juice. It has a salty flavor and can be used as a salt substitute. Kelp tablets should be taken as prescribed by your nutritionist. Dried kelp can be diced and added to soups and stews.

KIDNEY BEAN   This hard, red, kidney-shaped bean is rich in protein and vitamin B. There are white beans of similar shape that also fall under the same name but are sometimes called marrow or cannelloni beans. The nomenclature of beans is intricate! Try mixing the white with the red in this picturesque cold salad. See also *Beans, Dried*.

KIDNEY BEAN SALAD

    2 cups cooked red kidney beans
    2 cups cooked white kidney (cannelloni) beans
    1 medium-size red onion, finely chopped
    16 artichoke hearts

DRESSING:

    3 tablespoons olive oil
    1 tablespoon lemon juice or balsamic vinegar
    1 clove garlic, chopped
    1 teaspoon fresh oregano
    ½ teaspoon fresh dill weed
    Salt and pepper to taste

- Cook the beans in separate pots; otherwise the white ones will catch a dingy hue from the red. Mix the cooked and cooled beans, chopped onion, and artichoke hearts. Combine dressing ingredients and toss salad in dressing.
- When well mixed, refrigerate for at least 3 to 4 hours.
- Serves four to six.

KOMBU This seaweed (a type of kelp) is a very healthful plant, full of iodine and other minerals. It comes in thick green sheets that must be soaked before cooking, then cut into strips. Sauté with vegetables, add to soups, or sauté alone with tamari soy sauce as a seasoning.

KOMBUCHA The kombucha "mushroom"—which is actually a colony of yeast and bacteria—acts on the combination of sugar and black tea to produce this semisweet fermented beverage that hosts a variety of stunning nutritional claims. Popular in Russia, this fizzy drink may take some getting used to, as it has a distinctly fermented taste, but it is worth the effort, as kombucha is reputed to combat cancerous conditions, eliminate gallstones, detoxify the body, restore alkalinity, boost the immune system, aid in weight loss, control the appetite, cleanse the liver, and speed up metabolism. Health benefits aside, there is no denying the immediate jazz of energy that one feels after a good dose of kombucha.

For anyone who has tried to make their own kombucha, chances are a stab of guilty relief might have been experienced upon discovering the sudden arrival of the prebottled kombucha that has recently been appearing in the refrigerator section of many health food stores. Not that growing kombucha is that difficult. In fact, it is quite simple. However, because of its tendency to expand seemingly on a daily basis, kombucha does demand a certain level of care and attention, and it is quite easy, after only a couple of months of ownership, to have trouble finding room in the refrigerator for anything else. New batches must be made every few weeks, using a base of black tea, sugar, and a cup of kombucha from the previous batch, and from each batch comes the opportunity to separate out another "mushroom" and make another batch, which then makes another "mushroom"... with no apparent end in sight.

The kombucha "mushroom" can be purchased or acquired from a friend. Once begun, the kombucha mushroom grows layers at an astounding and slightly intimidating rate, and many kombucha growers are known to become kombucha pushers, as it can become nearly impossible to drink enough kombucha to be able to use all of the resulting "mushrooms." When one's friends tire of receiving, the compost pile often becomes the only option.

KUZU ROOT This tuberous root (also known as kuzu arrowroot and kudzu) has been grown in remote mountains of Japan for thousands of years and is supposed to have healthful qualities that tropical arrowroot lacks. In the late 1800s kuzu, which is a member of the legume family, was introduced to the United States. Like arrowroot, it is ground into a white powder and used as a thickener of sauces, soups, and gravies. Taken medicinally as a beverage, it is said to be an energizer and to give relief from colds and diarrhea, and it is high in protein, fiber, and vitamins A and D. The leaves and stems of kuzu can also be eaten, and have been a popular staple in both Japan and China for thousands of years.

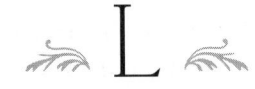

L

LECITHIN   Lecithin has long been used by the candy and baking industries as an emulsifier and a preservative. Baking industry aside, however, lecithin has nutritional value of its own and is said to reduce the cholesterol level in the body, to help eliminate liver spots, to be beneficial in cases of dry skin and psoriasis, to stimulate sexual vigor, to aid in some cases of arthritis, to stimulate brain activity, and so on. Quite enough to send one dashing out for a bagful of lecithin granules!

Lecithin is found in all nonhydrogenated oils, egg yolks, liver, and soybeans. It occurs in conjunction with that oft-discussed substance, cholesterol, and seems to be essential to its proper absorption. For it is far more important to absorb the cholesterol ingested than to try to bar cholesterol from one's diet. If you use hydrogenated oils—this includes commercial peanut butter and all margarines—or like to savor the fat on your steak and lamb chops, best to add some lecithin to your diet. The need for lecithin increases with age.

Lecithin used to be extracted from egg yolks; now it is most commonly taken from the soybean. It is available in granules that can be used like wheat germ or added to soups and stews and baked goods. One or two teaspoons a day is a usual dosage. Added to bread and other baking, it will act as a preservative: substitute one-third of the oil called for in any recipe with lecithin, at the rate of 1 tablespoon lecithin to 2 tablespoons oil.

LEMONGRASS   This grass is native to Southeast Asia, where it is considered to be one of the most important flavorings, specifically for Thai and Vietnamese dishes. The fresh stalks are about two feet long, greenish-gray, and resemble scallions in that they are bulbous at the tips. It is this bulbous white base that is thinly sliced and used to impart a distinctive lemon flavor to soups, sauces, and curry dishes, and teas. Lemongrass is tough and fibrous and should be removed from the dish before serving. Fresh lemongrass can be stored for up to two weeks in the refrigerator.

LENTIL, BROWN   One of the oldest of the leguminous plants, the humble lentil was cultivated by the ancient Egyptians and the Greeks. The lentil grows in pods like its botanical cousin the pea—there are two lentils in each small pod—and has long been known as a food of the poor people, for it offers its high protein far more cheaply than the rich man's beef. As a meat substitute, lentils are a valuable food in vegetarian diets, and in Catholic countries are much used during Lent. The protein contained in lentils, however, is not complete; therefore, a meal of lentils should also include some other source of protein—perhaps a sprinkling of nuts, hard-boiled eggs, or a little cheese. The husk of the lentil seed is sometimes rather difficult to digest, but this can be overcome by adequate cooking or by straining or blending the cooked lentils. It is said that the gas-producing tendencies of lentils are lessened if they are eaten with fruits or vegetables.

COLD LENTIL SALAD

2 medium onions, chopped

2 cloves garlic, chopped

11 tablespoons olive oil

2 cups dry lentils

4 whole cloves

2 bay leaves

Salt and pepper to taste

Water to cover

3 tablespoons balsamic vinegar

DRESSING:

½ cup Italian parsley, chopped

1 large onion, chopped

1 tablespoon Dijon mustard

Juice of 1 lemon

Salt and pepper

2-3 tablespoons olive oil (enough to thicken)

Sauté 2 onions and garlic in 4 tablespoons olive oil until transparent. Add all remaining ingredients except the vinegar and remaining olive oil and simmer until lentils are just cooked—do not overcook.

- Drain, remove cloves and bay leaf, and cool. Then toss lentils in 7 tablespoons olive oil and the balsamic vinegar.
- Mix dressing ingredients, except for olive oil. Slowly add oil until dressing thickens. Add to lentils and mix well. Garnish with watercress and tomato wedges.

MEATLESS PATÉ WITH BROWN LENTILS

1 cup brown lentils

1 cup walnuts, chopped and toasted

2 tablespoons butter

2 onions, chopped

2 cloves garlic, chopped

½ cup red wine

2 teaspoons dried thyme

1 teaspoon dried oregano

1 teaspoon basil

1 tablespoon Dijon mustard

Salt and pepper to taste

- Cook lentils in just enough water to cover, for 20–30 minutes or until tender. Add water if needed during cooking. Drain.
- Chop the walnuts finely and toast. While lentils cook, sauté onions and garlic in butter. Deglaze pan with red wine, and mix with cooked lentils, onion mixture, and remaining ingredients.
- Preheat oven to 350 degrees and oil a one-quart loaf pan.
- Bake the loaf for 30 minutes. Cool and remove from pan.
- Serves eight to ten.

LENTILS, FRENCH French, or green, lentils have a delicious subtle flavor. They hold their shape more readily than their brown or red counterparts, which lends an aesthetic elegance to their presentation. Considered by some to be the most nutritious and rich of the legume family, lentils are high in phosphorous, zinc, iron, calcium, potassium, and vitamin B complex. Try French lentils with a dollop of sour cream on top and a sprinkling of diced chives. Though simple in nature, few dinner guests will be disappointed by such tasty fare.

LENTIL, RED   The famed red pottage for which Esau sold his birthright was most likely made from the Egyptian red lentil. Today these tiny orange-red beans are also cultivated in northern France and are greatly valued for their delicate flavor. In Scotland the red lentil is also often used, and is sometimes known as "Scottish cereal."

Red lentils have a subtler flavor than their stalwart brown confreres. They cook quickly without presoaking, and can be used in soups, stews, and Indian dal.

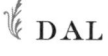 **DAL**

> 2 tablespoons butter
>
> 1 large onion, chopped
>
> 1 teaspoon salt
>
> 2 teaspoons turmeric
>
> 2 tablespoons ginger powder (or 1 tablespoon fresh, chopped)
>
> ½ teaspoon chile pepper
>
> 1 teaspoon cumin powder
>
> 1 teaspoon ground coriander
>
> 1 cup red lentils, washed and drained

- Sauté in butter all ingredients except lentils. When onions are soft, add 2 cups boiling water and the lentils. Lower heat and simmer covered for 20 minutes or until lentils are tender. More water may be added if a thinner sauce is desired.

- This dish will burn easily, so use a heavy pot and watch it carefully. Serve alone or as a sauce over rice, bulgur, or kasha. No proper Indian meal is ever complete without its dal.

- Serves four.

LICORICE ROOT   The bark of the rhizomes and roots of this perennial herb has been used since ancient times. Its sweet pungency has been extracted for making beverages, candies, and pastries. Try giving a child a stick of licorice root to chew on instead of the artificially sweetened conglomeration that now bears the name of licorice (yet which rarely contains any real licorice whatsoever). Use a licorice stick to clean your teeth.

As a medicinal, licorice root gives relief from sore throats and coughs. It is often an ingredient in throat lozenges. Add a few chips off a licorice root to some rose hips, and you will have a delicious tea that is extremely good for colds.

Licorice has a laxative tendency. Pregnant women should avoid licorice root, as should those with diabetes, high blood pressure, or liver or kidney disorders. To take licorice medicinally for more than four weeks at a time can be risky and lead to water retention, high blood pressure, and impaired kidney function. As with any medicinal herb, moderation is always a safe measure.

LICORICE ROOT
life size

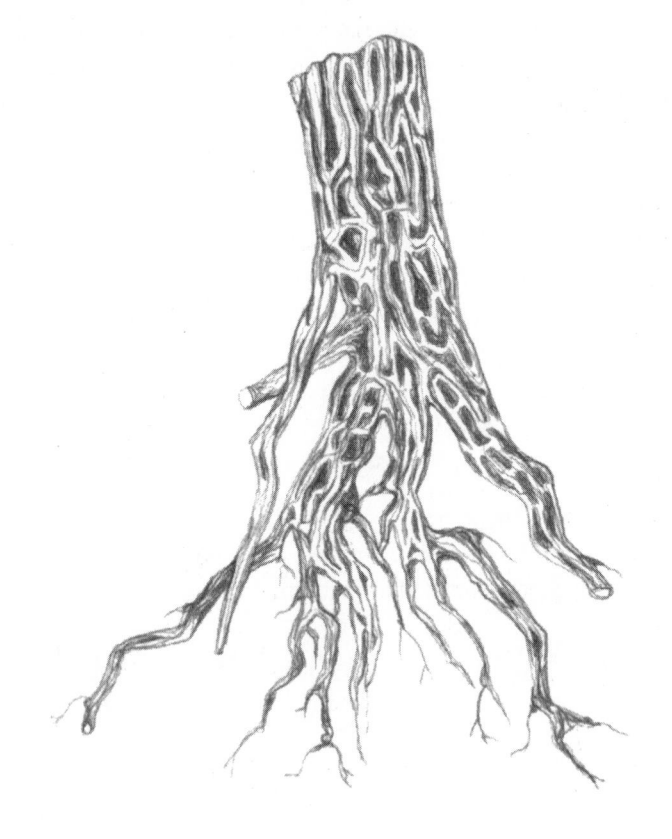

LINDEN TEA   The sweet-scented flowers and heart-shaped leaves of this tree have made it a symbol of love and a poetic subject for generations. The linden is also known in the United States as basswood. Both the flowers and the leaves are used in making a medicinal tea. Boil together in water, then strain and use either hot or cold. This infusion is very useful in promoting perspiration and is a good remedy for coughs and vomiting.

LINSEED OIL   Linseed oil is expressed from the linseed or flaxseed. When cold-pressed, it is relatively odorless and tasteless and may be used for cooking and salads. Widely used as a medium by painters and for making paints, varnishes, and linoleum, the commercial oil is extracted by use of high heat and is *not suitable for human consumption*. See also *Flaxseed*.

LOTUS ROOT TEA   This sweet and mild tea may be made from either the fresh or dried root of the Asian lotus plant. In either case it is said to be very helpful for respiratory problems. Fresh, the root is grated and boiled in an equal amount of water with a pinch of salt; strain and serve. The dry root, which is usually powdered, is prepared by mixing 1 teaspoon of the powder with 2 cups water. Simmer and just before serving add a bit of grated ginger and tamari soy sauce.

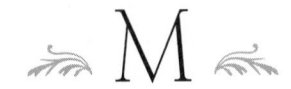

M

MACE   As the pear-shaped fruit of the nutmeg tree splits open with ripeness, a bright red filigreed network is revealed, which encases the nutmeg kernel. This network is mace. It is carefully removed from the kernel, dried (losing its red color for a rich brown), and ground for use as a delicate culinary spice. Mace can be substituted in any recipe calling for nutmeg; the taste of the two is quite different—and yet somewhat the same. Use mace in cookies, bread, and cheese; or to add flair to rice, ground meat, and fish sauce.

It is good to remember, however, that mace, as with nutmeg, in very large amounts can be dangerous and produce toxic results.

MALVA TEA   Also known as mallow, the leaves of this common wayside weed (*Malva rotundifolia* or *M. neglecta*) yield a tea that is high in vitamin A and minerals—a good tonic. The leaves also lend pungency and health to soups and salads. Poultices of the leaves can be used to treat insect bites and other skin irritations.

It would probably not be a good idea to gorge yourself on malva leaves, however—they have been implicated in some cases of livestock poisoning.

MANGO, DRIED   Besides being stunningly beautiful, both on the tree and off, mangoes have a sweet, juicy, delicate flavor unlike any other, a taste so delectable, in fact, that mangoes may be one of the most popular fruits on the market. It is said that Buddha was given the gift of an entire grove of mango trees where he could rest when he wished, a legend that has earned the mango the mythical value of being able to grant wishes.

Dried mango is a sweet and tasty treat that is high in vitamins A and C, as well as potassium and beta-carotene. Dried mango is at its best when organic and dried without the addition of unnecessary sugars. The result is an energizing, somewhat leathery piece of mango that is considered a delicacy by adults and children alike. As always, be sure to purchase only unsulfured dried fruit!

MAPLE SYRUP, PURE Pure maple syrup is, alas, a vanishing commodity. Imitation "pure" maple syrups abound on the markets; even those syrups claiming to contain no additives have usually been processed in a most distasteful manner. In 1962 the Food and Drug Administration sanctioned the use of formaldehyde tablets (or pellets) in the tap holes of sugar maple trees. Although this law was passed in the name of sanitation, the truth is that the tablet keeps the tap hole open and allows the sap to flow much earlier and longer than it should or ever has. The supreme flavor of syrup tapped at its prime is utterly lost. As for the formaldehyde, its users claimed that it evaporates as the syrup is boiled. We, however, would feel more at ease if the formaldehyde had kept its old-fashioned place on the poison shelf. Also, bacterial cultures may be added to the syrup to restore proper flavor, and antifoaming agents are often used. Though formaldehyde tablets are now banned, it is rumored that some disreputable maple syrup farms still use them. Know your sources and demand untreated syrup.

Yet after all is said and done, because the syrup is made by evaporation and is exposed to heat for a long period of time, the finished product is no more nor less than a delicious sugar. It might be more healthful to use unheated honey or molasses on your next batch of pancakes—but we cannot pretend that there is really any substitute for the delicate sweetness of pure maple syrup!

MAPLE MOUSSE

    1 pint heavy cream
    3/4 cup maple syrup
    6 egg yolks, beaten well
    Pinch of salt
    1/4 cup ground nuts

- Beat heavy cream until it is thick but not whipped. In a double boiler heat the syrup until it is just warm. Add egg yolks slowly, stirring constantly. Add salt. Stir until the mixture thickens—about 3–4 minutes.
- Remove from heat and stir until it cools. Fold in the cream. Pour into one larger bowl or into individual cups and put in the freezer of your refrigerator.
- Remove frozen mousse from the freezer 20 minutes before you plan to serve it. Sprinkle ground nuts on top. A luxuriously rich dessert.
- Serves six.

MARJORAM   Sweet marjoram is the more restrained relative of wild marjoram (oregano). Its name derives from the Greek for "joy of the mountain." Certainly it is a joy in the kitchen! It is particularly good (fresh or dried) with lamb and other meats and will lend delicious flavor to scrambled eggs and steamed vegetables. Its flavor is subtler than oregano's, but it nonetheless has a pungency to be reckoned with judiciously.

Marjoram, like many other herbs, was appreciated in prerefrigeration days for its disinfectant qualities. As a tea, it is mildly tonic, but other herbs are more medicinally inclined than this one. Its oil is used as a liniment to relieve neuralgia and sprains. Before the days of hops, it was used to brew beer and ale.

MARJORAM OMELET

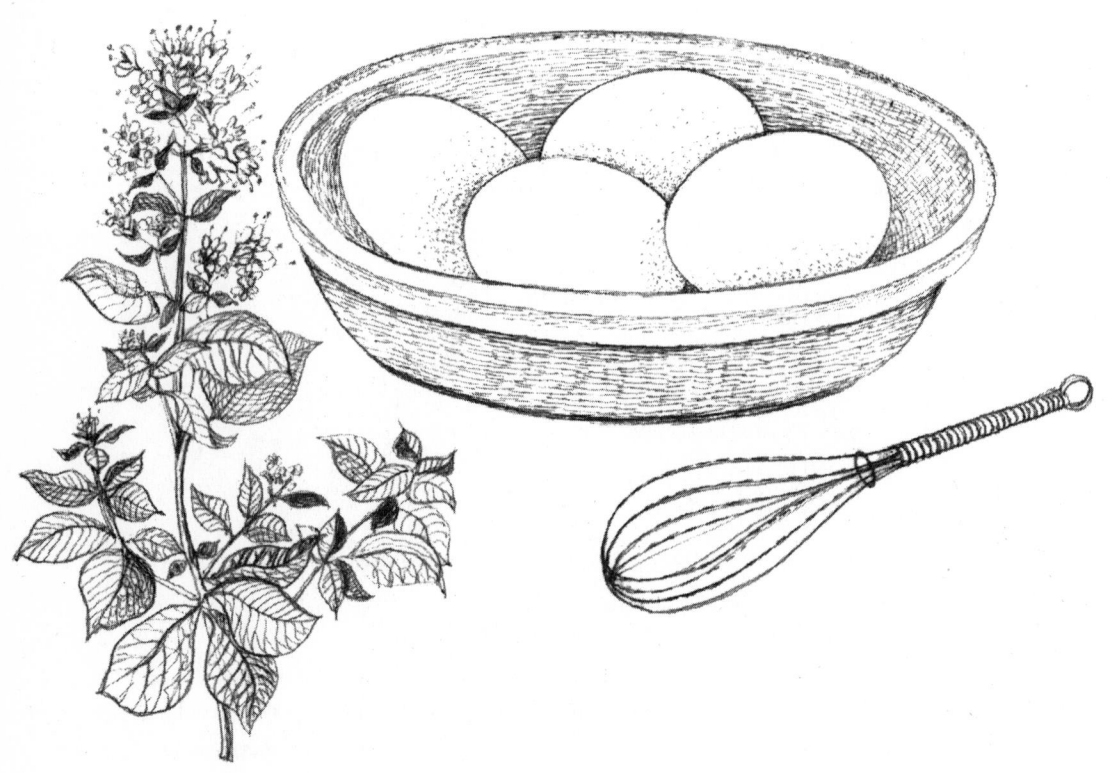

MARJORAM OMELET FILLING

3 cloves garlic, chopped

³/₄ cup fresh parsley, chopped (or ¹/₃ cup dried)

3 medium onions, sliced

1 tablespoon butter

2 tablespoons olive oil (preferably pressed oil)

5 cups sliced zucchini

1 teaspoon dried marjoram (or 2 teaspoons fresh)

¹/₂ teaspoon salt

¹/₄ teaspoon ground black pepper

Sauté garlic, parsley, and onion in butter and oil for 3–4 minutes—do not brown. Add zucchini, marjoram, salt, and pepper. Cook until tender. Set aside and keep warm while you make the omelets.

This makes enough filling for 4 two-egg omelets or 1 eight-egg omelet. Spoon the warm filling onto one side of the omelets (or omelet) while it is still in the pan; fold in half.

Serves four.

MARSHMALLOW ROOT   This geranium-like herb (*Althea officinialis*) grows wild along coastal salt marshes in Europe and the United States and can also be cultivated in your garden. The name usually brings to mind the white marshmallow confection, which was originally made from powdered root of marshmallow. Today's marshmallows, however, no longer have anything whatsoever to do with this very useful herb—being made as they are of a nutritionless conglomeration of corn syrup, sugar, and gelatin.

Powdered or pounded marshmallow root can be used as a poultice to ease skin irritations such as burns, bedsores, and abrasions. The sliced root can also be boiled to make a tea; it is said to alleviate hoarseness and coughs because of its emollient qualities.

An old saying has it that the marshmallow plant will only grow near happy homes.

MARSHMALLOW TEA   This tea is prepared with the leaves and flowers of the marshmallow plant (see *Marshmallow Root*) and has a number of beneficial uses—for lung and throat problems as well as for coughs and tender gums. It is also helpful in cases of dysentery and bowel inflammation. Applied to the eyes, the tea eases inflammation and sties; as a douche it soothes vaginal irritations. In all cases it functions, like the marshmallow root, as a softener or emollient, and as such alleviates discomfort rather than offering a cure.

To prepare the tea, simply take about 2 teaspoons of leaves and/or flowers and let them steep for 10 to 15 minutes. Strain and add honey if you like.

MEAT   The idea of a herd of beef cattle grazing on a grassy hillside on a warm summer day is delightful, but sadly not very realistic. Today a larger percentage of our cattle than anyone would care to admit are raised in the quickest, cheapest, least healthful, and most unnatural manner possible. Probably no food on the market is altered as much as meat. Nutrition and even the modicum of health—either of animal or of human consumer—are ignored, and money is the motivation in the meat-producing business.

Most beef cattle are now conceived through artificial insemination, immediately weaned on foods loaded with drugs, pesticides, antibiotics, and synthetic vitamins (so much for the old-fashioned virtues of mother's milk and verdant pastures!), and finally shot full of tranquilizers and meat tenderizers before being led to the slaughter. The woeful lives of unfortunate pigs, veal calves, lambs, and chickens follow the same maleficent pattern. Pigs are fed processed garbage; veal calves are kept in a state of acute anemia and absolute immobility in order to produce pale, muscleless meat; lambs may be shorn chemically, with the chemical then penetrating into the flesh, while "spring" lamb is now produced twice yearly by manipulating the light of an artificial environment; chickens are raised in windowless superstructures, with their arsenic-doused food (for yellower skin) passing by on conveyer belts. Other problems we are faced with in our meats are coloring to make the meat look fresher longer, and chemicals (such as cancerous nitrates and nitrites) to make it last longer without obvious spoilage. Commercially raised chicken is rife with salmonella and disease. Lunchmeats are thick with preservatives.

If you are not prepared to make the leap to organic meat for monetary reasons, there are certain precautions that can be taken to ensure more health and less contamination for you and your family. Choose your butcher carefully; find out where he gets his meat and how it has or has not been treated; watch to make sure the ground meat is freshly ground in a well-cleaned grinder; have as much fat as possible trimmed off the meat, for it is in the fat that the pesticides leave a great deal of their residue. There is controversy over whether liver is still fit for human consumption. Some contend that because the liver is the body's "clearinghouse," as it were, all of the chemicals the animal has been exposed to are deposited there in concentrated form. Others claim that the health value and vitamin B content of liver are so high that liver remains one of the healthiest of meats. For this reason it is supremely important to purchase both beef and chicken liver that comes from organically raised, antibiotic-free, free-range animals.

MILK, CERTIFIED RAW   Certified raw milk is unpasteurized milk that has to meet high and rigid standards of quality. The cows producing such milk must be fed fodder uncontaminated by pesticides, regularly inspected for disease, cared for by absolutely healthy personnel, and the equipment carrying milk from cow to container must be completely sterile. These rules are strictly enforced, and milk bearing the certified label is absolutely safe to drink and highly nutritious.

Pasteurized milk, on the other hand, is steadily declining in nutritional value and carries in it many harmful elements. Antibiotics that are pumped into cows in pasteurized herds go straight into the milk and are not killed by pasteurization. Neither are the pesticides nor the hormones eliminated. Bacteria count is allowed to be extremely high in the belief that pasteurization will kill everything—which somehow becomes like the difference between drinking boiled contaminated water and pure springwater. Pasteurized milk is often exposed to excessively high temperatures that destroy large amounts of its calcium (the main reason we drink milk!) and alters its nutritional content extensively.

If you cannot find certified raw milk—try to buy from a local farmer whose operation you know is clean. There are still a few regional dairies around that pride themselves on a particular herd of Alderney or Guernsey cows that are thoughtfully cared for. Search them out! Then you will be getting all of the rich vitamin A and D, potassium, phosphorus, calcium, and protein that you deserve from a glass of milk. If certified raw milk makes you nervous despite the strict regulations, then choose to buy only organic pasteurized milk, as this milk (though not as nutrient rich) will at least be free from the hormones and pesticide residues that contaminate all other dairy milks.

MILK, POWDERED NON-INSTANT   Skim or whole non-instant powdered milk has been spray-processed at a very low temperature and its nutritional value left more or less intact. It is high in protein, calcium, and minerals. Instant powdered milk, however, is heated at extremely high temperatures and thereby loses enormously in nutritional value. Instant powdered milk is also difficult to use in cooking and cannot be added directly to recipes without detrimental effects—bread becomes leaden and yogurt stringy, to give just two examples. Non-instant powdered milk, on the other hand, adds body and nutritional value to just about anything you care to add it to—gravies, cookies, soups, bread, yogurt, etc.

Powdered milk should not, however, be considered a complete substitute for fresh milk; its composition has been altered in the drying process, and despite all its benefits, it has become an unbalanced food. But as a fortifier of other foods, it is extremely useful. Make fortified milk by adding non-instant powdered milk to regular milk at the rate of ½ cup powdered milk to 1 quart fresh milk. Remember after opening powdered milk to keep it in a tightly sealed jar; moisture can cause its bacteria content to rise.

MILLET   Millet is probably one of our most ancient grains and has been used in India, Africa, and the Middle East since prehistoric times. Its name derives from the Latin *mille* (a thousand), referring to the prolificacy of the millet seed. This grain grows easily in a wide range of soils and climates, and a large variety of species fall under its name—ranging from sorghum to the small pearl-like grains that we know and eat as "common" millet.

Millet is a particularly nutritious grain, containing good amounts of iron, magnesium, potassium, and some protein. It can be used as a breakfast cereal, a rice substitute, or ground coarsely (a blender will do) and added to wheat flour for deliciously different loaves of bread.

Although millet is most commonly seen in the United States as an ingredient in birdseed mixtures, it deserves a place on your table as well.

MILLET PARMIGIANO

> 1 cup millet
> 2 cups boiling water (or broth)
> 2 tablespoons butter
> 1 teaspoon salt
> 3 tablespoons grated Parmesan cheese

- Toast millet in pot until it gives off a delectable nutty aroma, stirring to prevent burning. Add boiling water or broth, butter, and salt. Simmer in a covered pot for about 40 minutes or until water is absorbed and millet is soft. When done, fluff with a fork and sprinkle grated cheese on top.
- Serves four.

MILLET, CRACKED   Cracked millet falls between whole millet and millet meal in size and can serve as a substitute for either. Used in bread instead of meal, it gives a slightly crunchy loaf. When used as a main dish or cereal instead of whole millet, it is finer in texture and cooks more quickly. Try it as a cereal with toasted sesame seeds sprinkled and honey ribboned generously over it. See also *Millet*.

MILLET MEAL   Ancient Romans made their bread of millet meal and wheat flour. Try adding ½ cup ground millet (a blender or coffee grinder will do the trick if you cannot buy the meal commercially) per each 5 cups of wheat flour to your next batch of bread. See also *Millet*.

MINERALS   Minerals are inorganic substances found in food that are essential to human life. Ideally, all the minerals we need should be obtained from the food we eat. Often, however, they are lost in cooking or were never there in the first place, due to poor agricultural and processing practices. So mineral supplements are sometimes necessary. Minerals obtained from natural sources are far more easily assimilated than are chemically isolated minerals.

MINT   The mint family of herbs is a large one. There are more than twenty different species of mint and hundreds of related species. Apple mint, Indian mint, Bowles mint, horsemint, bergamot mint, pineapple mint, Corsican mint (which is used for making *crème de menthe* liqueur), even catnip (see *Catnip*), are a few of the many minty variations that can grow in your garden or lend aroma to your lemonade and tea. Mint is often mixed with various herbal teas to give added flavor. Peppermint tea stands on its own, with superb flavor and healthful qualities that work wonders on an upset stomach, promote digestion, and are soothing during times of colds and flu. Spearmint and peppermint are the two most widely used types of this herb (see *Peppermint; Spearmint*).

MINT BASMATI RICE WITH LEMONGRASS

    1 cup basmati rice
    2 cups water or broth
    2 tablespoons olive oil
    1 stalk lemongrass, very finely chopped (use innermost, bottom
        section)
    2 cloves garlic, finely chopped

1 tablespoon fresh grated ginger

2 tablespoons mint, chopped

- Bring water to a boil in a small saucepan. Add rice, reduce heat so that rice is simmering and cook, covered, for 20 minutes or until all the water has been absorbed. Meanwhile, sauté all other ingredients, except mint, in olive oil. When rice is done, add sautéed mixture. Sprinkle with fresh mint and serve.
- Serves two.

MISO   Miso is a dark soybean paste that has been aged in wooden barrels for three years. There are several types of miso: *mugi*, *hacho*, and *kome*. *Mugi* miso is for everyday use, particularly good for temperate weather, of medium strength, and made of soybeans, barley, sea salt, and water. *Hacho* miso is stronger in taste, good for cold weather, yang in tendency, and made from soybeans, sea salt, and water. *Kome* miso is the most mild in taste, particularly used in hot weather and for women and children, and is made from soybeans, brown rice, sea salt, and water.

Miso has a beneficial action on intestinal bacteria similar to that of fermented milk. Miso is also very high in easily assimilated proteins. Mix ¼ teaspoon miso with a little water and add to 2 cups hot water for an invigorating broth; add it to any soup for a bouillon flavor. Take care to add miso toward the end of the cooking, however, and do not boil it or some of its healthful properties will be destroyed. Miso can be used uncooked in dips and sauces and spreads. Here is a delicious sandwich filling.

MISO BUTTER

½ cup miso

Water

1½ cups sesame tahini

- Mix the miso with a little bit of water to make a smooth paste. Add tahini and blend well. Very good on a slice of dark whole grain bread. This will keep a long time refrigerated.

MOCHI   Native to Japan, mochi is made from glutinous rice that has been steamed, mashed or pounded, and then flattened. Mochi is available prepackaged in the refrigerator section of most health food stores. When baked, it is transformed from a dense substance to a puffy, pastrylike form that is crisp on the outside and extremely chewy on the inside. Mochi is available both plain and sweetened and makes a great snack food for kids.

MOLASSES

When sugarcane juice is boiled down and the raw sugar extracted, a thick dark syrup remains. This is blackstrap molasses. Further refining yields a slightly paler, less strong-tasting molasses. Both are highly nutritional, particularly compared to their devitalized relative, refined sugar. Blackstrap molasses takes the lead, however, in high iron, potassium, calcium, and vitamin B content. An extremely valuable substance in the treatment of iron deficiency, low energy, constipation, and nervous strain, its taste, however, is rather overpowering; but when mixed half and half with honey and used to flavor yeast drinks, cereals, bread, milkshakes, or yogurt, it is quite palatable. Do not take it straight from a spoon; it tends to stick to the teeth and may cause decay.

GINGERBREAD MEN

$\frac{1}{3}$ cup butter
1 cup molasses
$\frac{1}{2}$ cup yogurt
$\frac{1}{4}$ cup sugar
$3\frac{1}{4}$ cups unbleached white flour
$1\frac{1}{2}$ teaspoons baking soda
$\frac{1}{2}$ teaspoon ground cloves
2 teaspoons ground cinnamon
2 teaspoons ground ginger
$\frac{1}{2}$ teaspoon salt

- Preheat oven to 350 degrees. Lightly oil a cookie sheet.
- Cream butter and molasses together. Add yogurt and sugar. Sift in flour, soda, spices, and salt. Mix well; the dough will be fairly stiff. Roll out dough on a floured board and cut into gingerbread-men shapes, or form shapes with your hands without rolling out.
- Place on cookie sheet and bake for 12–15 minutes until lightly browned.
- Makes about two dozen.

MU TEA

Mu means infinity, and this tea is said to lead you up the road toward infinite wisdom. However that may be, mu tea is a delicious beverage. You may want to save it for special occasions, for it is very expensive. It is a mixture of sixteen exotic herbs and seeds: ginseng, ligusticum, herbaceous peony root, cypress, orange peel, ginger root, rehmannia, cinnamon, cloves, peach kernels, coptis, licorice root, cnicus, stractylis, moutan, and hoelen.

The tea comes in a small package that should be emptied into a quart of water and boiled about 20 minutes. Use an enamel pan—never aluminum. Strain and serve. The herbs may be saved and used one more time, but do *not* wait more than two days, or they will lose flavor.

MUGICHA BARLEY TEA   Made from roasted unhulled grains of barley, this tea has a rather strong taste and is used by some people as a coffee substitute that is very popular in Japan. Put a generous pinch in 2 cups water and boil for 20 minutes. Strain and serve.

MULLEIN BLOSSOM TEA   Make certain that your mullein blossoms are bright yellow, for therein lies their medicinal value. When carefully dried to retain their color, they can be a helpful aid against coughs, chest trouble, colds, and inflammations of the throat or mouth. Steep 2 teaspoons blossoms in 2 cups of boiling water until it reaches a summer yellow; drink as needed. Add honey for a tastier tea. The vapors of the tea may be inhaled and will relieve congestion due to colds.

Mullein blossom tea is occasionally referred to as verbascum, the generic name of the plant from which it is prepared.

MUNG BEAN   These small green beans are grown primarily in India—from whence comes their name—but they are also cultivated on a smaller scale in many other tropical countries. In America they are most frequently used to make sprouts that are sweet and crunchy, tender enough to be used raw, and substantial enough to stand sautéing. The sprouts are highly nutritious, contain large amounts of vitamin C, and are very simple to grow. For sprouting instructions, see *Sprouts*.

MUSHROOM, DRIED   Dried mushrooms are a delectable item that should be on every kitchen's shelf. Not only are they an epicurean delight; they are also rich in B vitamins, riboflavin, potassium, and phosphorus, and contain vitamin D and protein. They can of course be used to replace fresh mushrooms, but the dried mushroom should also be appreciated as a food itself. A wide variety are available; one can savor the vivid differences between Italian, French, and

Chinese fungi; whereas with fresh mushrooms we are often limited to the varieties offered by commercial markets.

Dried mushrooms give excellent flavor to soups, sauces, and stews. Before using, wash them, then soak in water to cover for 30 minutes. Do not throw out the brown soaking water; add it to your recipe for delicious additional flavor.

SAFFRON RICE WITH DRIED MUSHROOMS

1/4 cup dried mushrooms

2 cups liquid (water or broth and mushroom water)

1 teaspoon salt

1 cup basmati rice

1/4 teaspoon powdered saffron

1 1/2 tablespoons butter

1/2 cup grated Parmesan cheese

Pepper to taste

- Wash and soak mushrooms in water to cover for 30 minutes. Drain and save water. Slice mushrooms if they have become very large during soaking.
- Add mushroom water to broth or water to make 2 cups, add salt, bring to boil, and slowly sprinkle in rice so that boiling does not stop. Add mushrooms. Cover and simmer 20 minutes until rice is tender. Fold saffron into rice with fork until rice is evenly yellow. Then fold in butter, cheese, and pepper.
- Serves four.

MUSTARD   The seed of the robust mustard green contains a volatile oil that is a delight to the tongue but a problem for the innards—too much mustard can cause inflammation of the stomach and intestines. There are two varieties of mustard seed—white (sometimes called yellow) and black; black is the stronger. Whole mustard seeds are used in pickles and relishes. Ground mustard seed is said to have originated in the eighteenth century when a fine lady of Durham, England, thought to grind the mustard seed into a powder, discarding the husk. This "Durham" mustard caught the eye of King George I, so the story goes, and thence soared to popularity. Ground mustard is now widely used in sauces, salad dressings, and cheese dishes; or as a condiment in itself, mixed with water, white wine, or beer. Of the many varieties of prepared mustards available, Dijon and Dusseldorf types are generally considered to be the finest.

As a medicinal, mustard has long been in use, having received the endorsement of Hippocrates himself. The mustard plaster—made of equal parts ground mustard, flour, and water (add an egg white and additional flour when applying to very sensitive skin)—gives time-honored relief for congested lungs and muscular aches. Do not leave such a plaster on for too long, or it will cause the skin to blister. A sure—and not particularly pleasant—way to induce vomiting involves gulping down a glass of warm water with a teaspoon of mustard powder dissolved in it.

SWEET CURRIED CHICKEN

2 tablespoons curry powder

2 tablespoons soy sauce

½ cup prepared mustard (Dijon is good)

½ cup mild honey

1 (3-pound) chicken, cut in half or in pieces

- Mix together curry powder, soy sauce, mustard, and honey. Spread over chicken and marinate for ½–2 hours.

- Place chicken bone side up in 350-degree oven. Cook 30 minutes, then turn chicken over and baste so that a glaze will form over chicken; bake 30 minutes more, or until meat is tender. Serve with rice.

- Serves four.

N

NETTLE TEA   If you have ever been stung by the prickly leaves of this wild herb, you may be reluctant to think of the nettle as a food. However, when dried or boiled, nettles completely lose their sting; pick them with gloves and scissors, and you will be master of the situation. Boiled, they become a spinachlike vegetable, tasty and high in vitamin A, iron, and a wide variety of minerals.

Either the leaves or the roots of the common stinging nettle (*Urtica dioica*) may be used to brew a tea that has valuable powers as a tonic and blood cleanser, and it is extremely effective against kidney problems. When using dry nettle leaves, note that the greener they are, the more healthful.

A strong nettle tea, made by boiling a teaspoon of dried leaves in 2 cups water (or vinegar) for 30 minutes, is a very good hair rinse and is said to reinvigorate the hair and restore waning color. Slightly more obscure uses of nettle: beat rheumatic or paralytic limbs with nettle branches to restore vigor and circulation (this may also call for masochistic tendencies!); spin thread from nettle stems and weave table linen, as did the Scandinavians and Scottish in times of yore.

NONI JUICE   The fruit of the *Morinda citrifolia* has been used for centuries by the Polynesians, who recognized it as being of great medicinal value, as well as an indispensable food source during times of travel. The plant was spread from island to island, because the Polynesians traveled with noni fruit in their boats as they colonized the islands of the South Pacific. Considered to be one of the most beautiful plants in Tahiti, the *Morinda citrifolia* yields yellow and white fruit, roughly the size of a russet potato, year round.

Traditionally, Polynesians pick the noni fruit before it ripens, place it in a jar in direct sunlight, and then, when it is fully ripened, mash the noni into a purée and extract the juice through a cloth. Reputed to increase mental clarity, enhance immune function, increase energy levels, and support proper digestion and nutrient absorption, noni juice can be purchased in the nutritional section of many health food stores.

NORI   This Japanese seaweed comes in thin sheets, which are toasted quickly over the burner of your stove, then crumbled and used as a garnish over vegetables, rice, noodles, or used as a covering for rice balls or sushi. Nori has all the healthful qualities inherent in the mineral-rich seaweed family, which is said to be particularly useful for thyroid and prostate problems and to neutralize toxic substances in the body.

NUT (See also individual nuts)   Nuts are among the most nutritious of all foods. They contain relatively more protein than most other foods of plant origin and are therefore of great value as a meat substitute. They are also high in unsaturated fatty acids, B vitamins, and a multitude of minerals—phosphorus, iron, and calcium, in particular. Because of this load of nutrients, nuts should be eaten sparingly and chewed well. For greatest nutritive value and easy digestibility, eat nuts in their most natural form. This means nuts freshly extracted from their shells; shells that have not been gassed (for easier cracking), bleached (for uniformity of appearance), or dyed (who needs purple pecans and red pistachios?).

Once the shell is removed from a nut, it will quickly grow rancid unless refrigerated. Therefore almost all shelled nuts are treated in obnoxious manners to give them indefinite shelf life, and they should be avoided if possible. When you must buy shelled nuts, try to purchase them at a health food store that keeps them refrigerated. Also give a wide berth to roasted nuts. These are cooked at high temperatures that destroy much of the nutritive value; they are often saturated with hydrogenized oils used in the "roasting" process; and they are usually oversalted and sometimes even sugared. Roast your own nuts; it's easy and the taste is incomparable.

ROASTED NUTS

- On top of the stove: In a heavy iron skillet, place 1–2 cups fresh-shelled nuts. Raw cashews, pine nuts, and pumpkin seeds are particularly delicious when fresh roasted. Adjust heat to medium high, and stir nuts until they begin to let off their delicious aroma (about 10 minutes)—be careful not to over-roast. Sprinkle with sea salt (stir in 1 teaspoon pressed vegetable oil, and the salt will cling evenly to the nuts) if desired, and serve warm.

In the oven: Place 1–2 cups fresh-shelled nuts on a baking sheet. Place in a 350-degree oven. Every 5 minutes stir the nuts. In about 15 minutes their heady aroma will let you know they are ready—be careful not to over-roast. Sprinkle with sea salt if desired and serve warm.

NUTMEG   Nutmeg is the seed of a small pear-shaped fruit borne by the East Indian *Myristica fragrans*, or nutmeg, tree. The same tree also produces mace, the latticed network that surrounds the nutmeg kernel, and in itself a spice.

Nutmeg is easy to grate whenever a recipe calls for it, so for the most savory results buy your nutmeg whole. Many people keep a small grater and a few nutmegs in a closed jar, handy for use. Be sure to remove any white powder that may be clinging to the surface—that is lime, which is often used to keep the nutmeg dormant and insect-free, and it is not good for the stomach.

Nutmeg will enhance most any dish; try a dash in black bean soup, or on buttered vegetables, and in anything made with milk—baked custard, bread pudding, cottage cheese.

Oil of nutmeg, made by crushing the hard seed, is said to settle the stomach. A drop only, in a cup of herb tea, should do the trick. And should you yearn for a good night's sleep, try applying the fragrant oil to the temples as you settle into bed.

SPINACH PIE

Pie crust for one-crust pie

Zest of 1/2 lemon

3/4–1 pound fresh spinach

2 tablespoons butter

3 eggs

1 cup ricotta (or small-curd cottage cheese)

1/3 cup grated Parmesan cheese

6 tablespoons cream (or milk)

1/2 teaspoon salt

1/8 teaspoon freshly ground pepper

1/4 teaspoon freshly ground nutmeg

- Preheat oven to 375 degrees.
- Add zest to pie dough, roll out, and line a 9-inch pie pan with dough. Bake for 10 minutes.

- While this is cooking, wash very well and drain spinach and cook briefly in the water that clings to the leaves, just until it is wilted. Drain spinach well, chop, and mix with the butter.
- In another bowl beat eggs, then mix in ricotta, Parmesan cheese, cream, salt, pepper, and nutmeg. Stir in spinach and butter. Spread into the partially cooked pie shell and bake 30 minutes in 375-degree oven, until it is browned and firm to the touch. Serve warm. (This can also be baked without the time-consuming crust.)
- Serves four to six.

CARROT AND PARSNIP PURÉE

1½ pounds carrots, peeled and cut into large chunks

1½ pounds parsnips, peeled and cut into large chunks

½ teaspoon nutmeg

2–6 tablespoons butter

4 tablespoons vegetable stock, chicken stock, or cream, to thin

1–2 tablespoons brandy (if you wish)

Salt and pepper

- Steam vegetables separately. Purée together in a food processor or blender with nutmeg, butter, and stock or cream. Add salt and pepper. Serve hot. This may easily be made into a soup by adding more stock.
- Serves six.

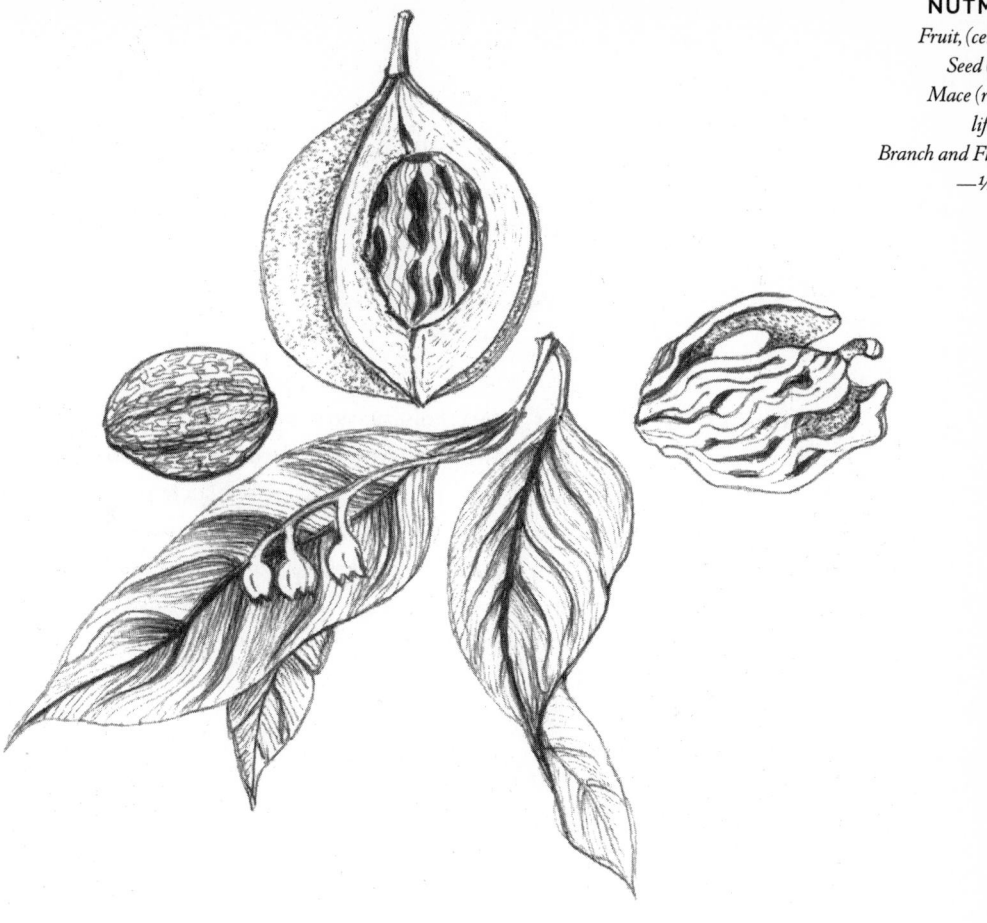

NUTMEG
Fruit, (center),
Seed (left),
Mace (right),
life size
Branch and Flower
—½ size

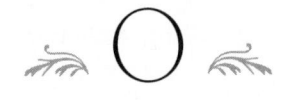

OAT FLOUR   Oat flour gives a moist sweetness to breads, pancakes, scones, and biscuits that is hard to match. This flour is also extremely good for the skin. Add to bath water and it will soothe the itch of irritations such as eczema, poison ivy, and poison oak. Or make a thick poultice of it with water and apply directly to the afflicted parts. These homemade preparations are just as effective and far less expensive than commercially sold "colloidal oatmeals." Oat flour is an effective skin cleanser and can replace soap when necessary; make a paste with water and apply to the skin, then rinse off.

OAT FLOUR SCONES

    1³/₄ cups oat flour

    ¹/₂ teaspoon baking soda

    2 teaspoons baking powder

    1¹/₂ teaspoons salt

    2 eggs

    2 tablespoons honey

    3 tablespoons sour cream

    2 tablespoons vegetable oil (or melted butter)

    1 tablespoon milk

- Preheat oven to 350 degrees.
- Mix oat flour, baking soda, baking powder, and salt.
- Beat eggs in another bowl, and set aside 1 tablespoon of egg to use for glaze. Stir in honey, sour cream, and oil. Add liquid mixture to dry mixture and stir well.
- Turn onto a board dusted with oat flour and knead briefly, using more flour if necessary. The dough will be soft and slightly sticky. Shape into a round ball. Place the ball on a lightly oiled baking sheet and pat out with hands into a

smooth circle; the dough should be about ½ inch in thickness. With a knife dipped in flour or cold water, cut the circle into 8 wedges, but leave them in place.

- ❧ Mix the reserved tablespoon of egg with milk and brush the mixture over the scones. Bake for about 30 minutes or until nicely browned.
- ❧ Makes eight scones.

OAT GROATS   Oat groats are the whole, uncut, uncrushed kernel of oatmeal. They can be used for cereal, but it's long cooking. They are most useful for sprouting and adding to salads and sandwiches. Oat sprouts are extremely high in vitamin B_2 and other valuable nutrients. See also *Sprouts* and *Oatmeal*.

OAT MILK   A common ingredient in face and beauty products, oat milk is good for more than just the skin. Oat milk is high in fiber, and vitamins A, D, E, and B, as well as a variety of healthful minerals such as iron, manganese, zinc, calcium, and magnesium. Introduced to the world by Sweden, oat milk is reputed to lower cholesterol if consumed on a regular basis.

OAT STRAW TEA   The leaves or straw of the oat plant can be simmered in hot water for 30 minutes and used as a tea that is said to be tonic, soothing, useful in treating allergies, and good for the heart and chest. The tea can also be added to your bath; it is good for sensitive skin.

OATMEAL   Oatmeal is a catchall term for any number of different types of oats. Steel-cut oats of various grinds, rolled oats, oat flakes, and oat groats may all be referred to as oatmeal. They are simply different treatments of the oat grain, which grows worldwide in climates that are too cold for wheat. Oats possess many healthful qualities—the celebrated physique of the Scots is said to be due to its virtues.

Processed oat products retain more of their original health value than processed wheat products; for when the oat is milled, the outer husk comes off but the bran and germ are left intact, unlike wheat, whose commercial milling removes both bran and germ. So you will get a better nutritional deal with the supermarket's rolled oats than with most other supermarket-type cereals. But still, they will contain pesticide residues and will probably have been exposed to excessively high temperatures to make them quicker cooking, which robs them of nutrients.

The "health food" version of rolled oats is usually called flaked or crushed oats, and the temperatures these products are exposed to are supposed to be low and carefully controlled to preserve food value.

With steel-cut oats you can hardly go wrong, for here the whole grain is merely sliced and otherwise untampered with. The finer the slicing of steel-cut oats, the quicker the cooking—it varies from 20 to 40 minutes depending on the degree of coarseness. Whole oats in pristine state (oat groats) take 1–2 hours to cook. Whole oats can also be sprouted (see *Sprouts*), resulting in an enormous increase in vitamin content, particularly vitamin B$_2$. Oat gruel (made by cooking and cooking and cooking whole oats until they become thick like a beverage) is said to be extremely healthful and was a popular drink in seventeenth-century London coffeehouses. Steel-cut and whole oats are slightly more difficult to digest than rolled, flaked, or crushed oats. All oat cereals encourage circulation and peristalsis and can act as a mild laxative. Oats are reputed to lower cholesterol and therefore to be good for the heart.

Leftover oatmeal need not be thrown to the birds. While it is still warm, mix in some raisins and hulled sunflower seeds, press into a buttered loaf pan, and refrigerate. The loaf can then be sliced any time, and the slices sautéed in butter—delicious with bacon and eggs. Or add leftover oatmeal to bread recipes; 1 cup oatmeal will replace about ⅔ cup wheat flour.

❧ OATMEAL PANCAKES

> 1 cup oat flakes (or rolled oats)
> 2 cups whole milk
> 1½ cups unbleached or whole wheat flour
> 1 teaspoon baking powder
> ½ teaspoon salt
> 2 tablespoons honey
> 2 eggs, beaten
> 4 tablespoons (½ stick) butter, melted

- Soak oat flakes in milk overnight in the refrigerator (if you give in and use commercial rolled oats, soaking is unnecessary).
- In the morning, mix flour, baking powder, salt, and honey into oat-milk mixture. Add beaten eggs and melted butter. On a lightly greased griddle, at medium-high heat, spoon small pancakes, cooking on first side until bubbly and then turning; try to turn each pancake only once.
- Serve with butter and honey or maple syrup. For other oatmeal recipes, see *Cereal*.
- Makes about 20 four-inch pancakes.

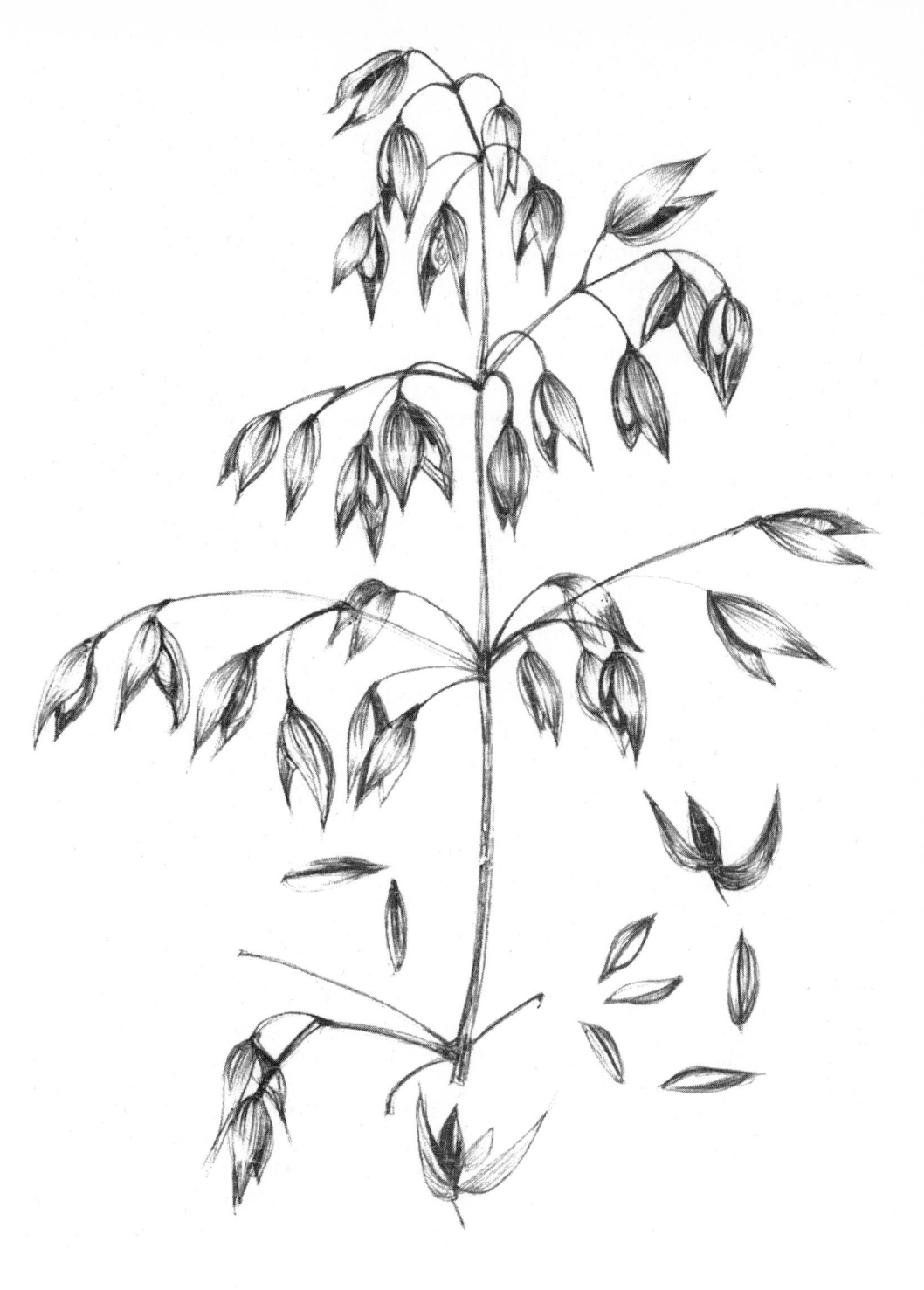

THE DICTIONARY OF WHOLESOME FOODS

GRANDMOTHER'S OATMEAL COOKIES

2 cups unbleached white flour

1 teaspoon cinnamon

½ teaspoon baking soda

½ teaspoon baking powder

½ teaspoon salt

1 cup (2 sticks) butter

1 cup sugar

2 eggs

4 tablespoons milk

1 cup raisins

2 cups steel-cut old-fashioned regular oatmeal (not instant)

1½–2 cups chopped walnuts or pecans

Preheat oven to 350 degrees. Sift dry ingredients together. In another bowl, cream butter and sugar. Add eggs one at a time, beating after each until smooth. Add milk. Add dry ingredients, then raisins, oatmeal, and nuts. Mix well. Dough will be stiff. Drop by the teaspoonful onto greased cookie sheet. Bake for 20–25 minutes.

Makes about two dozen cookies.

OATS, FLAKED   Flaked or crushed oats are similar to rolled oats, but are usually not exposed to such high temperature. They therefore retain most of their original nutritional value, but take longer to cook than commercial rolled oats. See *Oatmeal*.

OATS, ROLLED   These are oat kernels that have been hulled and flattened on steel rollers. They are often exposed to high heat, which lessens their nutritional value and makes them quicker to cook. See *Oatmeal*.

OATS, STEEL-CUT   Steel-cut oats are available in coarse or fine grinds. They are often known as Scottish oats, for in this form the Scots, who are centuries-old experts in the eating of oats, appreciate them most. See *Oatmeal*.

OIL, VEGETABLE   Vegetable oils occupy an important position in nutrition; it therefore pays to obtain the best quality available, even if it is somewhat expensive. How to recognize the "best" is a little tricky, but with a few basic facts under your belt you can surmount the problem with ease. First step: try to avoid commercial big-name brands. These oils are all extracted by use of petroleum-based solvents, and there is real danger of carcinogenic residues remaining in the oil. They are also exposed to excessively high heats and refining processes, which leave them odorless, tasteless, colorless—and unnaturally healthless. They are also permeated with preservatives. Stay away from them.

What you should aim for is a pressed oil in crude or relatively unrefined state. Pressed oils are obtained by use of hydraulic or expeller presses. The oil is forced by pressure out of the nut or seed or grain rather than being extracted chemically by use of solvents. Crude or unrefined oils are exposed to various degrees of filtration rather than to refinement by means of caustic chemicals.

Cast a wary eye on labels. Question the term "cold-pressed." All oil-giving substances (with the exception of olives and sesame seeds) must be exposed to a certain amount of heat before they will yield their oil. Question the term "unrefined." A truly unrefined oil is dark in color, thick in substance, and pungent in taste—and does not appeal to all palates. Question the term "virgin" (as in olive oil). As an indication of quality it is absolutely meaningless, for there are no standards governing its usage.

All properly processed vegetable oils provide excellent sources of unsaturated essential fatty acids, vitamin E, and lecithin. The type of oil you choose depends on your own taste or intention. Peanut oil is good for frying, and many Asian recipes blossom with it. Olive oil is unsurpassable for salads, and Italian dishes would lapse into lethargy without it. Corn, sunflower, and safflower oils are all highly unsaturated and good for general use. Then there are sesame, avocado, walnut . . . Experiment!

Always refrigerate vegetable oil after opening so that it will not become rancid. It will keep longer if it is in a dark container, for the oil deteriorates more rapidly when exposed to light. Vegetable oils can (and should) be successfully substituted for hydrogenated fats such as margarine, shortening, and lard in many recipes. Here, for instance, is an easy-to-make piecrust prepared with pressed vegetable oil.

🌾 PIECRUST

⅓ cup ice water

2 cups whole wheat pastry flour

1 teaspoon salt

⅓ cup cold butter

⅓ cup cold olive oil

- ➤ In a small bowl place an ice cube and about ⅓ cup water.
- ➤ Into a large bowl, sift flour and salt. Add cold butter, cut into small pieces. With fingers quickly mix with flour until butter and flour form pea-size lumps. Measure out ⅓ cup ice water and add ⅓ cup cold oil into same container. Pour all at once into dough and mix quickly with fingers, forming into a ball. Roll out immediately or refrigerate for later use.
- ➤ Makes enough pastry for one double-crust pie or two single crusts.
- ➤ *Note:* In order to have a flaky crust, the butter must not get too soft. Therefore work quickly; if at any point the butter seems to melt, refrigerate for a few minutes, then continue the recipe.

OLIVE OIL   The gnarled olive tree has been the purveyor of health and wealth since times of great antiquity. The Mediterranean shores were its earliest home, and in Homeric times olive oil was the luxury only of the very wealthy, who used it mainly as an ointment after bathing. Later in Italy, every single part of the olive tree found its use: the olive itself, ripe or unripe, as a delectable item of food; the oil as an adjunct to cooking; the oil as fuel for lamps; the oil as applied to the skin; the leaves and bark as a tonic tea; the resinous olive "gum" as a medicinal and perfume. During the heyday of the Roman Empire, a prescription for the pleasant life called for "wine within and olive oil without."

Olive culture has now spread to many parts of the earth, and California, China, and Australia have joined North Africa, Spain, France, Italy, and Greece as producers of olive oil. Italy remains, however, the high priestess of the olive, and little can equal the highest quality pure Italian olive oil. Olive oil varies tremendously in quality, depending on the type of olive used, the methods of refining, and whether it has been mixed with other cheaper oils. The term "virgin" is so widely and loosely applied that it no longer is any indication of quality; originally it meant that an oil was from the first pressing of the fruit, as opposed to the second or third pressings, whose oil is of inferior quality. Olive oil when unrefined has a greenish tinge and a very pungent flavor. It is preferred in certain areas to the refined oil, and certainly its healthful qualities are more intact—but you might have to cultivate a liking for the strong taste.

Olive oil oxidizes less rapidly than other oils; therefore, it does not need to be refrigerated to prevent rancidity. It is somewhat more saturated than certain other vegetable oils, but many a centenarian Italian has attributed his long life to the virtues of olive oil—and we side with the centenarians over the saturationists, and cherish our pure olive oil!

Use olive oil in cooking as you would butter. For a truly gourmet flavor, use half olive oil and half butter when sautéing or starting a sauce. Try sprinkling olive oil and lemon juice over hot vegetables, rather than the customary butter—it's delicious, it's healthy, and what is left over is great as a cold salad. Olive oil is incomparable in salad dressing. Here follows the way to dress a salad.

SALAD DRESSING
Have on your table:
A vial of pure olive oil
Sea salt
A vial of wine vinegar
A pepper grinder
A large bowl, no more than half-filled with freshly prepared salad

- Pour olive oil over the salad. (A quart of salad will take about 3 tablespoons oil, but this is variable; you want enough to coat all parts of the salad with a thin layer of oil, with none left in the bottom of the bowl.) Toss the oil into the salad until everything is well coated.

- Then put ½–1 teaspoon salt in a large spoon and fill spoon with vinegar (ratio of vinegar to oil should be about 1 to 3). Stir gently until the salt is dissolved in the vinegar, then sprinkle over the salad; add more vinegar if necessary. Grind pepper over salad. Toss well and serve.

- Salad should be served either before (health food style) or after (European style), never *with* the meal. With this method of preparing salad, the nutrients are sealed in by the oil so that the vinegar and salt cannot leach them out. The salad stays crisper, and salt, vinegar, and pepper are evenly distributed throughout rather than being deposited in clumps. Make a ritual of your salads!

OMEGA FATTY ACIDS   Omega oils are a family of fatty acids high in EPA, eicosapentanioc acid; DHA, dihomogammalinolenic acid; and GLA, gamma-linolenic acid, most commonly found in deep-sea saltwater fish such as salmon, mackerel, and tuna, as well as in flaxseed, evening primrose, and borage. Some of the long-term beneficial effects of adding omega fatty acids to your diet include smoother skin, lowering cholesterol, as a preventative against high blood pressure, and as an aid to preventing menstrual pain, migraine headaches, and depression. Omega-3 and omega-6 fatty acids are known to be essential for brain function, growth, and development.

Available in both liquid and capsule form, good quality omega oils should be found in the refrigerator section of the health food store, preferably in an opaque bottle, which ensures that the oil has been protected from light. Fish oil should be purchased only if it is of the highest quality, as many fish are not. If the fish oil leaves a lingering taste in the digestive tract, which it has been known to do, don't give up completely. Try an omega mixture of flax, evening primrose, and borage oil instead.

Want to sneak in a mental brain boost for the kids before they go to school? Try the delicious smoothie recipe found below, the kids won't even notice it's there and will most likely be clamoring for more. Filling and satisfying, an omega smoothie is the perfect way to start out the day. Trying to live a low-fat lifestyle? Remember, these fats are called "essential" for a reason, and when it comes to health, there are some fats the body simply cannot do without.

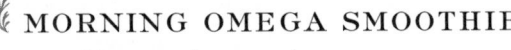 MORNING OMEGA SMOOTHIE

> 1 banana, frozen
>
> 5 strawberries, frozen
>
> 15 blueberries, frozen
>
> 2 tablespoons omega oil mixture of your choice, such as borage, flaxseed, and/or evening primrose
>
> $3/4$ cup grape juice
>
> $3/4$ cup apple or orange juice

- The best way to have frozen bananas on hand is to peel them, break them into one-inch pieces and freeze in a plastic bag.
- Toss all frozen fruit into the blender with omega oil of your choice, add juice, and blend. For a thicker smoothie, adjust juice accordingly. Experiment with different kinds of juice, coconut is great, as well as fruit combinations.
- Serves two.

OREGANO   Oregano, known also as wild marjoram and Mexican sage, is a hardy herb of the mint family. Its pungent flavor is often found in Italian, Greek, Mexican, and Spanish dishes. Use it sparingly, fresh or dried, or its taste will overdominate.

TOMATO-OREGANO SALAD

3 large cloves garlic

1 teaspoon dried oregano, or 2 tablespoons fresh

3/4 teaspoon salt

1/4 teaspoon freshly ground black pepper

3 tablespoons olive oil

1 tablespoon wine or balsamic vinegar

2 cups sliced fresh tomatoes

In a bowl press garlic cloves flat with the back of a wooden spoon. Rub oregano between hands to release oils and let fall into bowl. Add salt, pepper, oil, and vinegar. Stir and let sit for an hour or so. About 20 minutes before serving, add tomatoes, stirring to coat with dressing. Refrigerate briefly.

Serves four as a side dish.

TUSCAN MARINADE

6 cloves garlic, chopped

1/2 cup Tuscan olive oil

1/2 cup Italian red wine

1/4 cup fresh oregano, chopped, or 1 tablespoon dried

1/3 cup fresh sage, chopped, or 2 tablespoons dried

3 sprigs fresh rosemary, chopped, or 1 teaspoon dried

1 medium onion, chopped

1 teaspoon freshly ground black pepper

2 bay leaves

2 tablespoons orange or lemon zest

Combine all ingredients and refrigerate in a covered container. May be made up to four days in advance. Delicious marinade for steak or chicken. Marinate 2 hours before grilling, or overnight in refrigerator.

P

PANSY TEA See *Violet Leaf Tea.*

PAPAIN Papain, an enzyme extracted from the papaya fruit, is available in pill and powder form for use as a digestive aid. Papain has the ability to break down protein and is used commercially as a meat tenderizer. In tropical countries, natives obtain the same tenderizing effect by wrapping meat in papaya leaves or surrounding it with fresh slices of papaya fruit. See also *Papaya.*

PAPAYA, DRIED The mysterious and rich flavor of the papaya, which grows not on a tree but a large shrub, can be best appreciated when you are sitting on a sandy white beach in South or Central America. Should this be an impossibility, dried papaya is such a sweet and delicious treat that children just might accept a slice over a piece of candy. It is high in papain, a powerful digestive enzyme, as well as vitamins A and C. See also *Papain.*

PAPAYA LEAF TEA Papaya leaves contain papain, an enzyme that breaks down protein. The tea is therefore helpful in cases of indigestion and stomach disorder. It is often combined with peppermint, which strengthens its stomachic properties and gives it a delicious taste as well. Add 1 tablespoon dried papaya leaves to 2 cups boiling water and steep to desired strength. See also *Papain.*

PAPRIKA Paprika is made from finely ground sweet red peppers, which are rich in vitamin C. The many varieties of this spice range from very sweet to very hot. The paprika most commonly found in the United States is bright red and mild in flavor. True Hungarian paprika is of a more muted color and biting taste (there are, however, dozens of varieties and degrees of potency); if you are unable to find this, an approximation can be achieved by adding a tiny pinch of cayenne pepper to the tamer domestic paprika.

Paprika is used as a cheerful garnish on pale foods such as stuffed baked potatoes, egg dishes, and cold salads. It is a delicious seasoning in many fish, chicken, and meat dishes, and of course is imperative for Hungarian goulash.

PARSLEY   Put parsley in every dish you can think of. It is enormously healthful. It contains vitamins A and C in large quantity, along with chlorophyll, iron, and other minerals. Parsley's subtle taste complements almost every conceivable food. Use it fresh if possible. Flat-leaf or Italian parsley is tastier and tenderer than the conventional curly-leaf type. Parsley is a difficult herb to dry properly; when not carefully treated, it loses its color and its nutrients and becomes bitter in taste. Make sure your dried parsley is a healthy shade of green; that is an indication of good drying procedure.

Parsley tea, made by steeping 1 teaspoon dried leaves in 2 cups boiling water for 15 minutes, is said to be useful in the treatment of urinary tract infections, gallstones, and rheumatism.

PROVENÇAL POTATO SALAD

2 pounds small Yukon gold or red bliss potatoes (or a combination of both), halved

1 red bell pepper, seeded and thinly sliced

1 yellow bell pepper, seeded and thinly sliced

½ pound haricots verts (or string beans)

1 cup cherry tomatoes, halved

¼ cup capers

½ cup oil-cured black olives, pitted

3 scallions, chopped (use only white and pale green part)

1 tablespoon chopped fresh thyme

3 tablespoons chopped fresh parsley

DRESSING:

3–4 tablespoons red wine vinegar

9 tablespoons olive oil

1 shallot, finely minced

Salt and pepper to taste

🦃 Cook potatoes in salted water until just cooked. Drain. Put vinegar in a bowl. Slowly beat in oil. Add shallots, salt, and pepper. Toss warm potatoes with some of the dressing. When potatoes are cool, add remaining ingredients. Toss with more dressing.

🦃 Serves six to eight.

🌿 RACING STRIPE ASPARAGUS

2 pounds medium asparagus
2 hard-boiled eggs (preferably organic)
1 bunch curly parsley, chopped
4 tablespoons olive oil
2–3 tablespoons raspberry vinegar
Salt and pepper

🦃 Break off tough part of asparagus. Steam asparagus until tender. Do not over-cook. Cool. Peel eggs and separate yellow from white. Using the large hole of a four-sided box grater, grate egg yellow onto a plate. Then grate egg white onto another plate.

🦃 Beat olive oil slowly into the vinegar until blended. Add salt and pepper. Toss asparagus with vinaigrette. Lay asparagus lengthwise onto a platter. Then sprinkle a line of egg white across the stalks, followed by a line of parsley and then a line of the egg yolk, creating three colorful stripes!

PAU D'ARCO   Native to the rainforest and mountain ranges of Peru, Argentina, and Brazil, pau d'arco, also known as lapacho, is a tree that grows as tall as 120 feet and sports beautiful trumpetlike flowers that have also earned it the nickname Pink Trumpet Tree. It is the inner bark of this magnificent tree that has been used therapeutically for thousands of years.

Considered to have strong immune-building properties, pau d'arco is useful in fighting viral and fungal infections, as well as gastrointestinal upsets. High in antioxidants, pau d'arco is reputed to be helpful in treating arthritis, candida, herpes simplex, and yeast infections. Pau d'arco is available as a tea (it looks like finely shredded bark, but tastes mild and pleasantly nutty), a tincture, and in capsule form. Pau d'arco can also be used externally as a healing poultice.

PEA, DRIED   There are dried split green peas, dried yellow peas, and dried whole green peas—all rich in protein, sodium, potassium, magnesium, phosphorus, iron, and vitamin B. They provide the basic elements for extremely simple to make and satisfying soups. Whole peas are somewhat more time-consuming to deal with than split peas, for they have to be sieved to remove the tough outer husk that slips off while they simmer; they retain a higher food value, however, just because of this husky element. Split peas have been dehusked and split; dealing with them is simplicity itself, as you will see in the following recipe.

SPLIT PEA SOUP

2 cups split peas
2 quarts water
2 smoked ham hocks
1 bay leaf
Salt and pepper to taste

- Wash split peas well. Put in soup pot and cover with the water (use vegetable cooking water if you have it).
- Bring to a boil with the pot uncovered; skim off any foam that rises to surface. Turn heat low and add ham hocks and bay leaf. Cover and simmer for 2–3 hours, until peas have disintegrated and meat is so tender it falls off the bone. Stir well, add salt and pepper, and serve.
- Provides a sturdy meal for four.
- *Options:* Use ham bone or salt pork instead of ham hocks; or leave out ham altogether and add lightly sautéed fresh vegetables such as onion, celery, and carrots as the split peas begin to be tender.

PEACH, DRIED   Dried peaches are high in vitamin C, potassium, and phosphorus, and contain some vitamin B. When dried without sulfur and moisturizing treatment, they are tan and leather hard. Soaked and stewed with perhaps a little honey, they are delicious; put the stewed and sweetened peaches through a blender for a superb sauce to spoon over yogurt, cottage cheese, or ice cream.

PEANUT   The peanut is not actually a "nut" at all, but a member of the pea, or legume, family that grows in a most interesting manner. A rather low bushlike plant, it bears flowers that then become pods; the branches carrying the pods elongate, bend down, and push their pods into the ground; and when the plant dies, the mature peanuts (or ground nuts, as they are often called) are dug up.

Botanists are divided over whether the peanut came originally from Africa or South America. Now, however, it grows prolifically in almost all tropical countries; India and China are large producers, as is the southern United States.

Peanuts are a very nutritious food. They are extremely high in protein and unsaturated oil. Because their protein is incomplete, however, they should not be relied on as a sole source of protein. They are rich in vitamins E and B, particularly in niacin. The thin brown skin of the peanut contains trace minerals and B vitamins. Its slightly bitter flavor is appreciated by some, denounced by others. Shelled peanuts are available with or without this skin, so take your pick. Peanuts lose nutrients when they are roasted—but gain delicious flavor. It is best to buy raw peanuts and roast them in your own kitchen, for then you can control the temperature, the quality of oil, and the amount of salt used. Many commercially available roasted peanuts are actually deep-fried at high temperatures in low-quality oil and oversalted as well. To roast peanuts properly, place shelled nuts in a heavy frying pan over medium heat; stir until a roasted aroma arises; sprinkle on a few teaspoons of pressed oil, coating all nuts; stir in salt if desired.

Peanuts lend themselves to a wide variety of treatments—there is peanut oil, peanut meal, peanut butter, boiled peanuts, and roasted peanuts. Peanuts can be used as nutritious snacks or as part of a meal. Sprinkle crushed peanuts on salads; use them as a curry condiment, add them to soybean and grain dishes. Always buy peanuts organic, as they are known to have the highest levels of pesticide saturation among plant foods (besides the infamous raisin).

PEANUT BUTTER   The most popularly used "nut" butter in this country is that made from the peanut—usually the small variety known as the Spanish peanut. Because peanut-butter cravers run rampant hereabouts—and because many of them are children—it is important to realize the horrors that are perpetrated by the food industry on this highly nutritious comestible. Many commercially fabricated peanut butters contain as little as 75 percent peanuts. The rest is made up of hydrogenized fats (to prevent oil separation), sugar (for added sweetness and to mask the taste of inferior peanuts), emulsifiers (against oil separation), texturizers (to aid spreadability and counteract the butter's natural tendency to stick to the roof of the mouth), and degermed (for infinite shelf life) peanuts. Doesn't that sound appetizing!

Buy your peanut butter freshly ground and pure. Refrigerate during hot weather, and give it a stir before using, to redistribute the nutritious oils that rise to the top. Small trouble for the rich reward of delicious healthful peanut butter as it once was and still should be. See also *Peanut*.

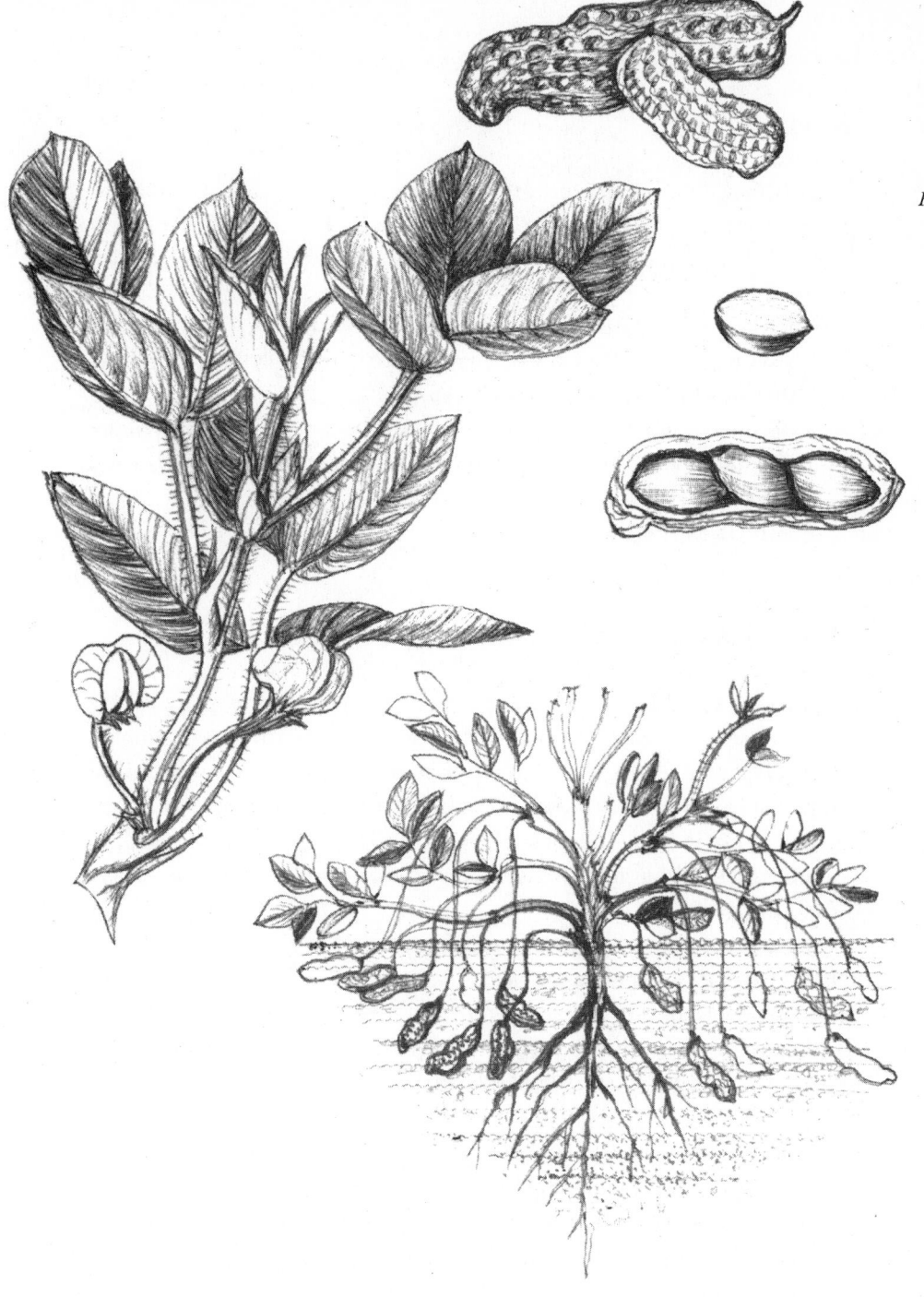

PEANUT
Plant—⅛ size
Fruits—life size
Flowers and
Leaves—
about ⅔ size

🌿 PEANUT BUTTER COOKIES

        1 cup pressed vegetable oil or butter
        1 cup peanut butter, unhomogenized
        1 cup honey or sugar
        1 teaspoon salt
        1 teaspoon baking soda
        2 eggs
        1 teaspoon vanilla
        2 cups whole wheat flour

- Preheat oven to 350 degreees. Lightly oil two cookie sheets.
- Mix oil and peanut butter. Add honey, salt, and baking soda, stir well. Add eggs and vanilla, then flour.
- When well blended, spoon onto the cookie sheet by the teaspoonful. Press down with a floured fork if desired. Bake for 10–11 minutes. Let cool on pan several minutes or cookies will crumble.
- Makes approximately 50 cookies.

PEANUT FLOUR   See *Peanut Meal.*

PEANUT MEAL   Peanut meal is made of finely ground peanuts. It is sometimes sold as peanut "flour." Like the peanut, it is rich in protein, vitamin B_1, riboflavin, and niacin. It can be used to boost the nutritional level of baked goods—and to lend delicious taste as well. Try using ¼ cup peanut meal to ¾ cup wheat flour in bread and cookie recipes. Use also as a substitute for chopped peanuts. This meal is available roasted or unroasted; the roasted type has a more distinctive nutty flavor.

PEANUT OIL   The peanut yields a light bland oil that is good for salads and cooking. It lends itself particularly well to frying, and is widely used in Asian wok cooking. Buy freshly pressed peanut oil, filtered rather than refined, without antioxidants, preservatives, and solvents.

PECAN   This native North American nut is delicious and healthful. It is thin-shelled and easily cracked. Buy pecans in their shells whenever possible. Out of the shell they will keep fresh only under refrigeration (unless preservatives have been added). And avoid the garish red-dyed pecans that appear in the markets these days; the dye rubs off on the hands and goes thence to the mouth. Pecans are naturally a pleasing brown color.

The pecan has a higher percentage of unsaturated oil than most other nuts and is rich in minerals, protein, and vitamin B. Because of its high content of vitamin B_6, it has been used in the treatment of neuritis and arthritis. Remember that the pecan is a highly concentrated food, and eat with a measure of restraint (though it is often difficult!). Pecan meal is easily made by grinding these tender nuts in a blender and can be added to bread and cookie recipes for a nutty flavor and nutritional boost; pecan meal is also easy to digest.

PECAN CRUNCH PEAR PIE

> Pastry for 9-inch piecrust (see piecrust recipe in book)
> 1 cup well-chopped pecans
> 7 firm pears, peeled and sliced (6 cups)
> 3 tablespoons mild honey
> $3/4$ cup whole wheat flour
> $1/3$ cup raw or brown sugar
> 1 teaspoon cinnamon
> 6 tablespoons butter

- Preheat oven to 375 degrees.
- Prepare pastry and place in a 9-inch pie pan. Sprinkle $1/3$ cup pecans over the dough and press in lightly. Chill the pastry while you prepare the filling and topping.
- In a large bowl combine the pear slices with honey and 2 tablespoons flour. Mix to coat all pears with honey and flour. In another bowl, combine the remaining flour and pecans with the sugar and cinnamon. Add butter cut into small pieces, and rub the mixture between your fingers until it forms pebble-size crumbs. Turn the pear mixture into the pastry shell and sprinkle the crumb mixture evenly over the top.
- Bake until the pears are tender and the topping is browned—about 40 minutes. Serve warm or cool.
- Serves six to eight.

PENNYROYAL   American pennyroyal (as opposed to its cousin, European pennyroyal) is an herb belonging to the vast mint family. It makes a flavorful tea, which is therapeutic as well—good for treating colds, constipation, headaches, sleeplessness, and delayed menstruation. American Indian women drank pennyroyal tea as a birth control measure. The herb is most useful as an insect repellent; grow it by your door to repel mosquitoes, or by the doghouse to scare the fleas, or put the dried leaves in closets to ward off moths. Pennyroyal leaves rubbed on the skin may protect you from insects. For tea, steep 1 tablespoon leaves in 2 cups boiling water; strain and serve.

PEPPER, BLACK The peppercorn, long grown in tropical Asia, was the main instigator of the profitable spice trade that grew up between the Far East and Europe. In the Middle Ages, Venice and Genoa waxed rich on its revenues; and even earlier, in the fifth century, the Visigoth king Alaric demanded 3,000 pounds of pepper as part of the ransom for Imperial Rome.

Peppercorns grow on vines in clusters of bright red berries. To produce black pepper, unripe berries are picked and sun-dried; the outer skin turns black and hard. Black pepper is widely used to flavor an enormous variety of dishes. It can be irritating to the stomach and intestines and is usually well avoided by those with ulcerous conditions. For those who can appreciate this pungent spice, always grind peppercorns fresh. There is really no excuse for using preground pepper; the difference in taste is incomparable.

PEPPER, GREEN This type of green pepper is not the familiar garden vegetable but the fruit of the *Piper nigrum* plant that yields black and white peppercorns. Green pepper is picked while unripe, and instead of being dried (which yields the hard black peppercorn) it is packed right away in vinegar. The resulting spice is green in color, soft in texture, and subtly pepperish in flavor.

PEPPER, RED Red pepper is the fruit of an extremely varied group of plants known as the *Capsicums*. They are native to tropical America and the West Indies and range in taste from sweet and mild to pungent and fiery hot. They are rich in vitamin C and have certain medicinal qualities (see *Cayenne Pepper*). Red pepper is prepared for cooking by grinding or chopping the dried pepper. Cayenne, paprika, and chili powder are familiar forms of this spice.

PEPPER, WHITE White pepper, like black pepper, is the fruit of the *Piper nigrum* vine that was originally native to India and is now widely grown throughout tropical Asia. White pepper is made from ripe, bright red peppercorns, which are soaked to remove the outer coat, then dried, leaving a pale tan hard peppercorn. White pepper is slightly less biting than black and is used primarily to

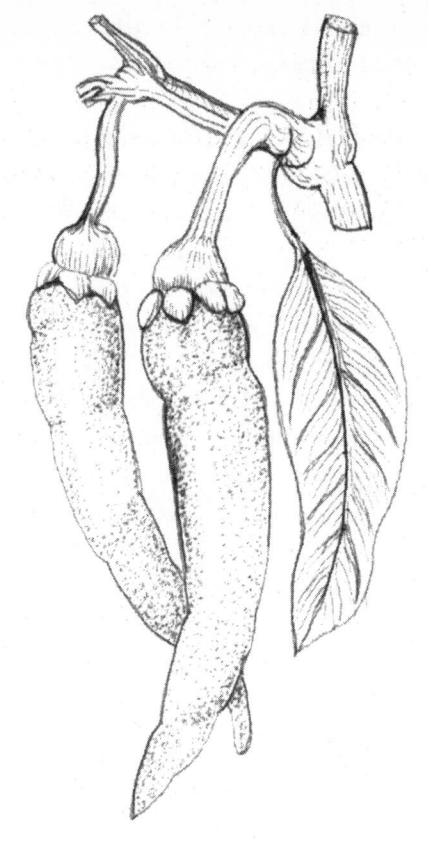

flavor light-colored sauces. Like black pepper, it should be freshly ground for superior results.

PEPPERMINT   Peppermint leaves (fresh or dried) are used primarily for making tea. Its tantalizing flavor and healthful qualities make it excellent for young and old … and those of us in between. Brew 1 tablespoon leaves in 2 cups boiling water until desired strength is reached. Add honey and lemon if you like, and drink for pure enjoyment, or for relief from colds, headaches, indigestion, and nervousness. Peppermint tea is very soothing after an attack of vomiting and takes away the bad taste. Peppermint is rich in vitamins A and C. When buying bag "peppermint teas," be sure that the content is pure peppermint leaf as opposed to orange pekoe tea with the addition of a few peppermint leaves.

Oil extracted from the peppermint leaves has long been used as a flavoring in toothpastes and mouthwashes, chewing gum, and candy. Peppermint oil is a useful item to keep in the medicine cabinet, for it will alleviate toothache when applied to a bothersome tooth. It will also act as a mild anesthetic in cases of surface burns, and a dozen drops in a cup of herb tea may waylay attacks of diarrhea.

PIGNOLI (PIGNOLIA, PINOLO, PINE) NUT Except in rare Italian markets, this soft buttery nut is always sold preshelled. That is because its "shell" is a tough solid pinecone, full of sticky resin and dozens of tiny pignoli nuts, each encased in its own hard covering. It is a difficult and messy business to get the nuts out, and not a job that most of us would like to tackle. The high price of pignoli nuts is due to these extraction problems.

Pignoli nuts are imported from the Mediterranean regions. They are very high in protein (though, like the peanut, this is not a complete protein), unsaturated fats, and minerals. Their delicate taste and soft texture make them suitable for use in a wide variety of dishes; add them to fish, vegetables, or spaghetti sauce. These nuts are used for cooking and not for snacking, and a few will carry you a long way.

Other varieties of edible pine nuts are found in Switzerland, Mexico, and the Himalayan regions. In the southwest United States and Mexico, the piñon tree produces nuts that are very similar to the pignoli (see Piñon Nut).

❧ SPINACH WITH PIGNOLI AND RAISINS

    1½–2 pounds fresh spinach
    2 tablespoons pressed olive oil
    2 tablespoons pignoli nuts
    2 tablespoons raisins
    Salt and pepper to taste

❧ Wash spinach very well and cook it in the water clinging to its leaves, until just tender. While it is cooking, warm oil over medium-low heat in a saucepan, add pignoli and raisins, and cook for 2–3 minutes.

❧ Put the cooked spinach in a bowl and toss with warm pignoli mixture and salt and pepper.

❧ Serves four.

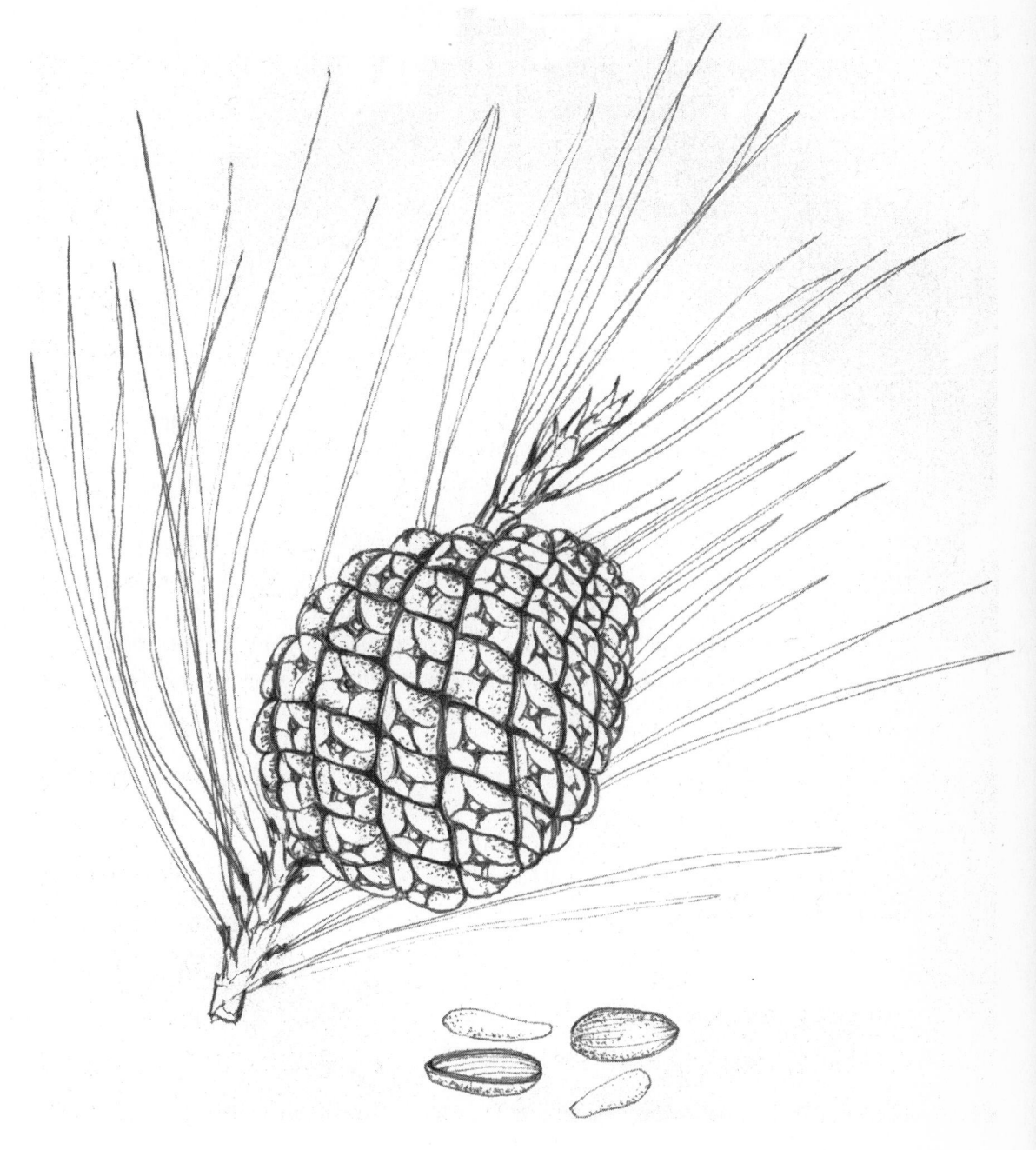

❦ HERBED CHICKEN WITH PIGNOLI

1 medium-size chicken

9 tablespoons olive oil (preferably pressed oil)

2 tablespoons butter

2 bay leaves

1 teaspoon dried rosemary (or 2 teaspoons fresh)

1 teaspoon dried sage (or 2 teaspoons fresh)

2 cloves garlic

1 teaspoon salt

$\frac{1}{4}$ teaspoon freshly ground black pepper

$\frac{1}{4}$ teaspoon grated nutmeg

$\frac{2}{3}$ cup dry white wine

2 tomatoes, peeled, seeded, and chopped

3 tablespoons pignoli nuts

❧ The chicken should be cut in pieces, washed, and well dried. Place oil, butter, bay leaves, rosemary, sage, and garlic (crush the cloves first with the back of a wooden spoon) in a pottery casserole or a Dutch oven. Sauté until the garlic just starts to brown.

❧ Put in chicken, and brown it over medium heat on both sides. Add salt, pepper, nutmeg, and wine. Simmer for 5–8 minutes, turning and stirring the chicken until the wine has practically evaporated and the sauce is quite thick.

❧ Add tomatoes and pignoli and cover the pot. Simmer gently for about 20 minutes. Then remove the top, and continue to simmer while the sauce thickens—about 5 minutes. Serve on top of egg noodles or polenta.

❧ Serves four.

❧ *Note:* This recipe also works well with a rabbit if there are no chickens handy.

❦ SUMMER PASTA

8 cloves garlic, chopped

Olive oil, approximately 3 tablespoons

2 pounds tomatoes, chopped (cherry tomatoes are great in this)

$1\frac{1}{2}$–2 cups fresh basil, chopped

$1\frac{1}{2}$–2 cups fresh mint, chopped

10 ounces feta cheese, cubed

$1\frac{1}{2}$ cups pignoli nuts, toasted

1 pound angel hair pasta, cooked
Salt and pepper to taste

- Sauté garlic in 1 tablespoon oil and mix with tomatoes and herbs. Add feta and pignoli nuts. Toss pasta with 1 tablespoon olive oil, and then add sauce and toss. Drizzle with remaining olive oil; add salt and pepper.
- Serves six.

PINE NUT See *Pignoli Nut.*

PINEAPPLE, DRIED The flowers of this tropical plant produce hundreds of tiny fruits that coalesce to form the single pineapple. Rich in vitamin C, with some A and B and assorted minerals, pineapples also contain a digestive enzyme similar to that of the papaya. Therefore, fresh pineapple, pineapple juice, and dried pineapple are all good for the digestion. Dried pineapple also makes a flavorsome snack.

PIÑON NUT The low-lying piñon tree grows in the southwestern United States and produces small pinecones that enclose the piñon nuts. These are very similar in taste and appearance to the pignoli nut of the Mediterranean, but they are far easier to extract from their cone. Piñons are not widely marketed, however, due mainly to the irregular productivity of the tree.

PINTO BEAN This tasty speckled bean thrives in the hot arid weather of the Southwest and Mexico. It is a good source of incomplete protein, amino acids, vitamin B, and minerals. The full flavor of pinto beans is best obtained by overnight soaking and long, slow cooking—4 hours of simmering will do, but if you can leave them to bubble gently on the back of the stove all day, so much the better. Use 3–5 cups water to every cup of beans.

Pinto beans, which incidentally lose their spots with cooking, are used in soups, stews, cold salads, and the Mexican frijoles refritos (refried beans).

PISTACHIO NUT If you have never tasted an undyed pistachio nut, you have a treat awaiting: a plain tan pistachio with a green-skinned kernel, lightly roasted and salted—unsurpassable! These nuts are particularly high in iron, vitamin A, and protein, with sizable quantities of potassium, magnesium, phosphorus, and vitamin B. Pistachios grow on small trees that are native to Asia and the Middle East; they are now cultivated throughout the Mediterranean region and also in the southern United States. These nuts are most often found in Middle Eastern confections and in ice cream.

POMEGRANATE JUICE   Some scholars now believe that it was actually a pomegranate depicted in the Garden of Eden, as opposed to an apple. One of the first cultivated fruits, even discounting the Garden of Eden, pomegranate trees were being planted sometime between 4000 BC and 3000 BC. Mohammed advised his followers to eat pomegranate, for it purged the system of hatred and envy.

Reputed to have higher antioxidant levels than any other juice, pomegranate is said to be helpful in the treatment of heart disease, in lowering cholesterol and blood pressure, for treating bladder infections, to aid in the expulsion of intestinal worms, and to relieve constipation. The dried bark and skin of the pomegranate is extremely astringent and is an ancient remedy for tapeworm. It will also give relief from diarrhea.

Pomegranate juice is undeniably an expensive treat (small wonder, considering how difficult they are to eat!), but so wonderfully healthful and delicious it seems well worth the investment. Pomegranate juice contains all of the pleasure of pomegranate, without the work.

POPPY SEED   The beautiful poppy flower owes its notoriety to the opium that is obtained from the flower pod. The seeds, however, contain no morphine, although a tea made from poppy seeds is said to have mildly calming properties. Poppy seeds can be either black or white; the black are of higher quality and white seeds are sometimes dyed to pass as black. They have a delicious nutty flavor and are widely used to flavor breads, bagels, and pastries. Try adding a teaspoon of poppy seeds to melted butter and pour over cooked vegetables—lends intriguing flavor.

The poppy seed also yields a bland light-colored oil. It has been used in parts of Europe for salads and cooking, and as an adulterant of olive oil. It is also serves as a medium for oil painting.

POTATO FLOUR   Potatoes did not enter the international cooking scene until the sixteenth century, when Spaniards in Peru came across Incas eating this all-American vegetable. The potato was enthusiastically adopted in Europe. By the nineteenth century the economy of Ireland had become so dependent on the potato that a failure of the potato crop brought the famine that started an enormous migration of Irish to North America.

Potato flour (also known as potato starch) is made of the entire cooked, dried, and ground potato. It is a very useful item to have in the kitchen. An ideal thickener for sauces, gravies, and soups, it cooks quickly and smoothly, leaving no raw taste (as wheat flour has a tendency to do). One teaspoon of potato flour will do the thickening work of 3 teaspoons of wheat flour. Potato flour can serve as a binder for ground meat and vegetable patties. It can also be used in bread making to condition the dough and to give added nutrients (potato flour is rich in vitamin C, potassium, and iron); as much as one-quarter of the wheat flour in any bread recipe can be replaced with an equal amount of potato flour.

PROTEIN   Proteins are necessary to maintain all forms of life—plant, animal, and human. They are complex substances made up of amino acids (twenty-two are needed by the human body; eight of them essential) and are indispensable to the building, growth, and repair of human body cells. They play an immensely important role during pregnancy, lactation, and childhood; it is absolutely necessary to ingest adequate protein at these times. Inadequate amounts can result in permanent body and brain damage.

The American diet has tended to emphasize meat as its prime source of protein. It is perhaps the easiest way to be sure of getting adequate protein, but there are many reasons to look for one's protein elsewhere—meat today is often tainted with additives and pesticides, and from moral or nutritional points of view it is distasteful to some people.

A vegetarian diet successfully requires a good amount of nutritional knowledge. Do not undertake vegetarianism lightly. For it is not only the quantity of protein that is important but also the quality; many plants contain incomplete proteins that must be properly matched with just the right companion plant or the protein is of little use to the body.

Prime sources of protein are meat, fish, eggs, milk, cheese, soybeans, brewer's yeast, some nuts, and wheat germ. Beans and many seeds and nuts are high in incomplete protein. There are any number of powdered protein supplements on the health food market. They have their place, perhaps; but there seems no reason why with a modicum of knowledge and planning one cannot obtain adequate protein in a more pleasurable and interesting manner!

PRUNE   Prune manufacturers valiantly attempt to rise above their constipation stigma. Cannot this fruit of the elegant plum tree stand on its own merits? For what is a prune but a dried plum—rich as it is in vitamin C, potassium, and protein. And delicious to boot.

Unsulfured, unmoisturized, unsugarcoated, unsprayed, sun-dried prunes are often so hard as to need soaking or stewing before savoring; be certain not to discard the juice—it is mineral-rich. Prunes are nutritious and good for the digestion; that they happen also to be efficacious in times of constipation seems superfluous to add.

❦ STEWED PRUNES WITH CINNAMON STICKS

     1 cup dried prunes
     2 cinnamon sticks
     4 cloves

    ❧ Place all ingredients in pot and fill with water to cover. Simmer 30 minutes, until soft. Serve over oatmeal, granola, or yogurt.

    ❧ Serves four.

PSYLLIUM SEED   Psyllium seeds supply bulk and lubrication to the intestinal tract and are used in conditions of constipation. Psyllium seeds can be chewed, in the fashion of the ancient Greeks, or added to cereal or blended into vegetable drinks.

PUMPKIN SEED   Pumpkin seeds (also known as pepitas) are crunchy and delicious, raw or roasted. Serve as a between-meal snack, or with cocktails, or toss them in with your fried rice. They are extremely rich in phosphorus, iron, and niacin and contain a good amount of protein, calcium, zinc, and other B vitamins, as well as omega-3 fatty acids. Renowned for their therapeutic effect on the prostate gland, pumpkin seeds are also said to destroy parasitic worms in the intestinal tract.

If you save the seeds from your next pumpkin, you can prepare them for eating: Dry them well for a few weeks, then peel off the tough outer skin. The inner kernel is edible either raw or roasted. This shelling process can be tedious; some pumpkins have seeds that are easier to handle than others.

❦ ROASTED PUMPKIN SEEDS

     1 cup raw pumpkin seeds
     ½ teaspoon vegetable oil
     1 teaspoon salt

Put pumpkin seeds in a heavy frying pan over medium heat. Stir in oil, coating all seeds lightly. Sprinkle in salt. Stir continuously until seeds are puffed up (be prepared for some to pop right out the pan!) and browned—this takes only a few minutes. Incomparable taste!

Q

QUINOA This "grain" (quinoa is not truly a grain, but the seed of a leafy plant) is native to the Andes and was cultivated and eaten by the Incas thousands of years ago. Quinoa flourishes under rough conditions, surviving drought, frost, and poor soil, and yet still manages to produce a high-protein seed with more calcium than milk and an abundance of amino acids, including lysine. Quinoa is reputed to increase milk flow in nursing mothers.

Though most quinoa is imported from South America, it is now being cultivated in the Colorado Rocky Mountains, where the conditions can be harsh enough to keep the quinoa growing well. A small yellowish grain with a sproutlike tail, quinoa cooks quickly to form a light, fluffy, and creamy dish. Quinoa has a bitter coating, called saponin, that protects the seed from predators and shields it from direct sunlight. The saponin has been removed before it reaches the store. However, quinoa should always be rinsed well before use in order to remove any remaining residue. Quinoa can also be ground and used as a nutrient-rich flour in breads and other baked goods.

QUINOA SALAD

1½ cups quinoa

1 small zucchini, diced

1 small carrot, diced

1 small red bell pepper, seeded and diced

1 small yellow squash, diced

5 tablespoons olive oil

2 tablespoons red wine vinegar

1 tablespoon chopped fresh tarragon

Salt and pepper

6 ounces goat cheese

- Cook quinoa in 3 cups of salted water, covered, over medium heat, until all water is absorbed (15 minutes).
- While quinoa is cooking, toss vegetables together. Make vinaigrette with olive oil, vinegar, tarragon, salt and pepper. Toss vegetables with cooked, room-temperature quinoa. Add vinaigrette. Toss. Crumble goat cheese on top.
- Serves four.

R

RAISIN   Raisins are dried grapes. They are mineral-rich and a good between-meal food for children—particularly tasty mixed with a few sunflower seeds. Try to obtain raisins from a reputable health food source. Commercially "sun-dried" raisins may be doused with insecticides and are known to have the highest pesticide levels of any other plant food besides the peanut! "Golden" raisins are usually treated with sulfur dioxide to preserve that golden color. Raisins are often moisturized by added water, to create that plump appearance, rather than by a careful drying process.

Use organic raisins in cereals, desserts, and bread. Or in this carrot salad.

CARROT-RAISIN SALAD

¼ cup lemon juice

½ cup raisins

1 tablespoon fresh parsley

2 cups grated carrots

¼ teaspoon prepared mustard

2 tablespoons mayonnaise (see recipe in book)

Salt and pepper

* Soak raisins in the lemon juice. While the raisins are soaking, chop the fresh parsley and grate the carrots. As soon as the carrots are grated, mix in the lemon juice and raisins to prevent discoloration. Add mustard, mayonnaise, salt, and freshly ground black pepper.

* Serves two as a main luncheon dish, or four as a side salad.

❦ PORTER CAKE

1 cup (2 sticks) butter, softened

1 cup soft dark brown sugar

2 eggs, beaten

1½ cups baking raisins

1½ cups unbleached white flour

3 teaspoons baking powder

½ teaspoon ginger

½ teaspoon cinnamon

⅛ teaspoon mace

½ cup Guinness stout

TOPPING:

¼ cup dried cherries, chopped

¼ cup raisins or dried cranberries, chopped

¼ cup nuts (walnut, pecans, or hazelnuts), chopped

½ cup apricot jam, warm

- Preheat oven to 300 degrees. Grease and line an 8-inch pan with parchment paper.
- Cream together butter and sugar. Beat in the eggs, a little at a time. Stir in the raisins, then fold in the flour, baking powder, and spices. Stir in the Guinness gradually until a smooth batter is formed. Turn into the prepared baking pan.
- Bake for 2¼–2½ hours until golden and firm to the touch. Cool, then turn out and wrap in greaseproof papers. Store for 2 days before eating. When ready to serve, mix dried fruit and nuts with warm jam to coat. Drizzle remaining jam over cake if desired, and top with fruit and nut mixture.
- Serves six to eight.

RED CLOVER TEA   The familiar pink-purple flower heads of the wild clover produce a tea that is high in vitamins C and B, calcium, potassium, and magnesium. An excellent tonic, and a blood purifier, red clover has a delicate taste; add a few peppermint leaves for a heartier flavor. Red clover tea is useful in the treatment of menopause, irregular menstrual cycles, and persistent coughs.

Red clover tea is also said to be quieting to the nerves. Gathering your own red clover sounds like a nerve-quieting activity, too! Dry the flowers in a dark airy spot and store in covered jars for winter use. To brew, steep 2 tablespoons blossoms in 3 cups boiling water for 10–15 minutes. Strain and serve with honey or lemon if desired.

RED RASPBERRY LEAF TEA   It should come as no surprise that a plant as delicate and delicious as the red raspberry would have medicinal value as well. In this case it is the leaves of the raspberry plant that are an indispensable addition to any tea cupboard. Recognized by Cherokee women to be vital during pregnancy, red raspberry is reputed to quell nausea, ease labor and delivery, and speed postpartum recovery. Because of its abilities to relax and tone the uterus, red raspberry leaf not only helps during birth and afterward, but it also aids in reducing menstrual cramps and normalizing hormones, while the tannins help to reduce excess menstrual bleeding. Reputed to relieve diarrhea, promote fertility, to relieve sore throats, and reduce fever.

Red raspberry leaf is rich in nutrients, including calcium, iron, B vitamins, manganese, and magnesium. The tea is flavorful and is a delicious alternative for pregnant women who are missing black tea, as the flavor of red raspberry leaf is reminiscent of a caffeinated tea, and it goes quite well with milk and honey. Red raspberry leaf can also be taken as a tincture.

Wild raspberry leaves are better than those of the cultivated varieties, but both are beneficial. If you gather your own leaves, make certain that they are completely dry before using; wilted berry leaves are said to be slightly poisonous. Raspberry leaf tea is also mildly laxative.

REJUVELAC   Originally created by Ann Wigmore, the pioneer of the "living food diet," rejuvelac is rich in enzymes and acts as an excellent fermented tonic, said to be cleansing for the intestines and colon, as it provides a source of friendly bacteria that are known to create healthy intestinal flora. Rejuvelac can be purchased at some health food stores in the refrigerated juice section or made at home.

HOMEMADE REJUVELAC

2 cups organic soft wheat berries
1 quart water

- Soak the wheat berries for eight hours to overnight. Drain through cheesecloth, rinse the berries and allow to sprout for two days in a jar with the lid covered with a cheesecloth.
- When white sprout tails begin to show, add water, cover the jar again with the cheesecloth, and place in a warm place for two days. Pour off the liquid rejuvelac and refrigerate. The rejuvelac is now ready.
- Rejuvelac should be cloudy, slightly yellowish in color (almost like fresh lemon

juice), and slightly carbonated. Drink, and store the remainder in the refrigerator.

- ❧ Temperatures higher than 85 degrees increase fermenting time, causing the rejuvelac to brew faster. In this case, reduce fermentation time. Lemon and honey can be added in order to increase palatability. A second batch can be made by refilling the jar containing the wheat berries and soaking for 24 hours.
- ❧ Makes one quart.

RICE, ARBORIO   This pearly, round, Italian rice is the foundation for cooking risotto, a dish that seems to exist solely as an example that Italians can make even the simplest ingredient, in this case rice, into a gourmet extravaganza of flavor. Arborio contains a higher than average amount of soluble starch, which is released during cooking, resulting in risotto's thick, creamy texture.

Grown in the Piedmonte and Lombardia regions of Northern Italy, risotto, like polenta, demands that the cook stand diligently over the hot stove for 20 minutes, stirring and adjusting. The resulting dish, however, is well worth the sweat on the brow and the aching wrist, and, chances are, dinner guests will be clamoring for a repeat performance.

RICE, BASMATI   Easily identified by its aromatic scent, the finest basmati rice is cultivated in India and Pakistan. Basmati, which means "fragrant" in Hindi, is available in both brown and white and complements curries and Indian dishes particularly well. Always buy organic, and rinse before using, as this will eliminate some of the rice's starchy residue and allow for a less sticky rice once cooked.

🌾 CHICKPEA AND BASMATI RICE SALAD

6 cups basmati rice

1 red bell pepper, seeded

1 yellow bell pepper, seeded

1 carrot

3 cups chickpeas, fresh cooked or canned

6 small scallions, thinly sliced, including part of the green

2 tablespoons sesame seeds, toasted

6–7 tablespoons sesame oil

2-3 tablespoons cumin

7 tablespoons lemon juice

5 tablespoons olive oil

Salt and pepper

- To cook basmati rice: bring 3 cups water to boil, add 2 cups of rice; lower heat and simmer 20 minutes or until water is absorbed. Fluff with a fork and set aside (or in refrigerator) to cool. Seed and chop peppers, grate carrot. Toss together the chickpeas, cooled rice, peppers, carrot, and scallions in a large bowl.
- To make the vinaigrette, stir together the sesame seeds, sesame oil, and cumin in a medium bowl. Whisk in the lemon juice. Slowly whisk in the olive oil. Toss the vinaigrette with the salad and season with salt and pepper to taste.
- Serves ten.

RICE, BHUTANESE   This red rice, which is native to Bhutan, a country nestled in the Eastern Himalayas, is so widely used in its own country that little is available to export. Bhutanese rice is well worth seeking out, however, as it has the same nutritional qualities as brown rice and yet cooks as quickly as white rice. Another reason to give this distinctive rice a try is that it demands little or no fertilizers or pesticides in order to be cultivated successfully, making the final product clean and healthy; it is said to be irrigated with thousand-year-old glacial waters, a process that also endows the rice with trace minerals. With a rich, nutty flavor and a soft texture, Bhutanese rice is best served with ingredients that have assertive flavors and will not be drowned out by such a robust accompaniment.

RICE, BROWN   An Asian grain that has been grown in India and China for more than 4,000 years, rice is a relative newcomer to the Western world. Its cultivation was not taken up in Europe until the fifteenth century and in America until the late seventeenth century.

Brown rice is the title given to rice that retains its healthful bran layer. Organically grown brown rice is not treated at any stage with insecticides, additives, or poisons. It is carefully milled, so that the bran layer and germ are unscratched, and this covering provides a natural preservative for the living grain beneath it.

Although brown rice is slightly lower in protein than various other grains such as wheat and millet, it is nevertheless highly nutritious and an excellent source of B vitamins. Macrobiotics consider it the most balanced and valuable of human foods. Its versatility in cooking can hardly be matched. An infinite variety of soups, stews, risottos, breads, and desserts can be built around a cupful of rice grains.

Brown rice is generally classified as short or long grain, and many regional variations exist within each group. Short-grain rice is considered to be slightly more healthful than long grain. All brown rice requires patient cooking—45 minutes to 1 hour. How much salt, how much water, how much time—all these are variable, depending on what your type of rice is, what kind of pot you use, even what the weather is like. Experiment, using the following recipe as a guide. Once you savor the flavor of brown rice, you may never want white rice again!

BROWN RICE

  2 cups water (for long-grain rice, try 2½ cups)
  1 teaspoon salt
  1 cup brown rice

- Put salted water in a heavy covered pot and bring to a rolling boil. Meanwhile place rice in a sieve and hold under cold running water, stirring it with your fingers. Again with fingers, sprinkle rice slowly into the boiling water so that the boiling does not stop. When all rice has been added, lower heat to simmering. Put a well-fitting cover on the pot and simmer for 45 minutes to 1 hour.
- If the rice is cooked too fast, it will burn at the bottom; if cooked too slowly, it will be soggy. Keep it at a slight bubbling simmer. The rice is ready when all the grains are tender but still separate; at this point the water should all be absorbed. If it is not, remove the cover of the pot, turn heat very low, and fluff with a fork until liquid is evaporated and absorbed. Add butter, or tamari soy sauce, or chopped herbs. From here on it's up to you!
- Serves two to three.

RICE, GLUTINOUS Known also as sweet rice, glutinous rice cooks to a rather sticky consistency and is used in Asia for dessert dishes. It contains less starch than regular rice and is also available in flour form.

RICE, JASMINE Officially known as Thai Hom Mali Rice, jasmine rice is native to Thailand. Similar in aroma to basmati rice, though milder, jasmine rice has a light floral taste. Light and slightly sticky, jasmine rice goes well with any Thai or Vietnamese dish.

RICE, KALIJIRA   Sometimes referred to as the prince of rice, Kalijira rice has only recently become available in the United States. A small, long-grained white rice, Kalijira is grown in Bangladesh. Similar to basmati, but in miniature, this petite grain takes only ten minutes to cook and has a delicate texture and aroma. Traditionally served using aromatic spices such as cardamom, cinnamon sticks, and cloves. Kalijira rice works well as a pilaf or as a stand-alone side dish.

RICE, SWEET   See *Rice, Glutinous.*

RICE, WHITE   By white rice, we mean refined or polished rice—rice whose vitamin-B-rich, beriberi-preventing bran layer has been removed, along with the germ; rice that has been treated with preservatives because its naturally protective outer coating is no longer around; rice that has been fumigated to give it long shelf life.

This processed rice is usually grown from seeds treated with toxic substances to make them disease-resistant, with the "help" of insecticide-sprayed soil chemicals to control weeds and water weevils, copper sulfate to control algae, parathion to control mosquitoes and larvae, and synthetic fertilizers. The straw and stubble and husks are all burned (yielding air pollution) rather than used to refertilize the earth. The result is a contaminated, nutritionally dead, starchy substance. But it is so white, so fluffy, so easy to prepare, that hordes of Americans find it impossible to resist.

For a healthful tasty alternative, see *Rice, Brown.*

RICE, WILD   Wild rice is the seed of a tall aquatic grass native to North America; genetically it is not a rice at all. It is delicious, expensive, and difficult to harvest. Native Americans harvest and sell much of the wild rice that is commercially available, often harvesting the grains by hand. Wild rice grows in many other parts of the country as well—often planted as a bird food by game hunters—but rarely does anyone bother to harvest it.

Wild rice has a much higher protein content than brown rice and is also higher in iron and phosphorus. Delicious in any setting, wild rice is a particularly fitting accompaniment for game and is often used in stuffings. Wild rice can be mixed half and half with regular rice for a dish that is easier on the pocketbook and yet exotically flavorsome.

RICE BRAN   Rice bran is made from the outer husks of the rice grain. We owe its existence to the fact that many people eat white refined rice—which leaves a rich "waste" full of vitamin B, calcium, phosphorus, and potassium. Use rice bran as you would wheat germ: Sprinkle on cereal and yogurt; add to baked goods.

RICE CREAM   This is a roasted brown rice flour that is used for making cereal or thick broth. You can make your own by toasting brown rice in a heavy frying pan, then grinding it to a powder in a blender, and re-roasting it over medium heat. Store in a tightly covered container and use as needed. Ideal for thickening, too.

SESAME–RICE CREAM CEREAL

> 2 cups milk
> 1 teaspoon salt
> ½ cup rice cream
> 2 tablespoons roasted sesame meal (or seeds)

Add salt to milk and bring to boiling point. Sprinkle in the rice cream, stirring to prevent lumping. Turn heat very low and cook covered for 5–10 minutes, until it thickens, stirring occasionally. Add the sesame seed meal. Serve with milk, butter, and honey.

Serves four.

RICE FLOUR, BROWN   Rice flour is a nonallergenic food and a great addition to a gluten-free diet. Brown rice flour, which is milled from polished brown rice, can be added to soups, baked goods, and casseroles for added fiber content and can be used as a thickener for sauces and gravies. This fine flour makes an ideal first cereal for babies and is deliciously smooth, mild, and less likely to cause stomach upset when compared to the more traditional cream-of-wheat baby cereals. Rice flour is sometimes sold under the name of rice cream.

RICE FLOUR COFFEE CAKE

> 2 cups rice flour
> 4 teaspoons baking powder
> ½ teaspoon salt
> 4 tablespoons sugar
> ½ cup raisins
> 1 tablespoon lemon zest

2 eggs, well beaten

1 cup milk

2 teaspoons vanilla extract

TOPPING:

4 tablespoons ($\frac{1}{2}$ stick) butter

4 tablespoons honey

$1\frac{1}{2}$ teaspoons cinnamon

- Preheat oven to 350 degrees. Butter and 8-inch square shallow baking dish.
- Sift flour, baking powder, and salt into a mixing bowl. Stir in sugar, raisins, and lemon zest. Beat together in another bowl the eggs, milk, and vanilla. Add to the dry mixture and stir until batter is smooth.
- On the stove, melt butter and stir in honey and cinnamon. Remove from heat and beat in egg mixture. Pour batter into prepared baking dish. Dribble topping all over the surface of the batter. Bake for 30 minutes. This is a light, moist cake, ideal for breakfast, afternoon tea, or dessert.
- Serves six.

RICE GRITS Coarsely ground brown rice grains—or grits—are good for hot cereals and puddings, and wherever the fluffy texture of whole rice is not required. They are also quick to cook.

RICE MILK Made from rice, water, and sweetener, rice milk is a great alternative for lactose-intolerant individuals. Useful in baking and over cereal or in tea, rice milk has a light refreshing quality that goes well with pancakes or just by the glass. Keep in mind that rice milk has a consistency similar to non- or low-fat milk and does not have the creamy texture many coffee and tea enthusiasts desire for their hot beverages. Rice milk is available both fresh and boxed and is often fortified with nutrients.

RICE MILK

4 cups hot water

1 cup cooked rice (warm), white, brown, or basmati will do, |experiment for a favored flavor

1 teaspoon vanilla

- Blend mixture until smooth. Let mixture set for about thirty minutes, then, without shaking, strain milk through a cheesecloth into another jar, allowing the sediment to remain in the original jar to be disposed of, preferably in the compost pile. Sweeten as desired.

⤚ Makes 4–4 ½ cups fresh rice milk.

RICE POLISH   The inner bran layers of the rice grain—known as the polish—are a by-product of rice refining. Rice polish is rich in vitamin B and minerals, but slightly less so than the bran that comes from the outer layers of the grain. Use as you would rice bran or wheat germ.

RICE SYRUP, BROWN   Made by adding sprouted rice or barley to cooked brown rice, brown rice syrup has a delicious butterscotch flavor. Full of complex sugars, which absorb more slowly into the bloodstream, a quality that inhibits dramatic shifts in blood sugar levels. Brown rice syrup is about half as sweet as cane sugar and can be added to baked goods in place of cane sugar.

ROOIBOS   Grown exclusively in the Cedarburg Mountains of South Africa, rooibos has been gaining popularity. Often identified as "red tea," the leaves of the rooibos bush are harvested, chopped, wetted, and left to ferment in heaps, then dried in the sun, a process that changes the previously green leaves to the stunning red color that we witness in our teapots.

Reputed to help in cases of hay fever, asthma, allergies, insomnia, infant colic, and stomach upsets, rooibos is caffeine-free. Try rooibos topically for the healing of acne, eczema, diaper rash, and even for stubborn cases of infant cradle cap. Rooibos contains flavonoids, which are free-radical-fighting antioxidants that are also found in green tea. However, the flavonoids in rooibos are said to be far more effective than those in green tea, which, combined with its caffeine-free status, makes rooibos a healthy tea worth keeping in the cupboard.

ROSE HIP   The hip of the rose is the urn-shaped seed receptacle at the base of the blossom. When the flower is in bloom, the hip is green. After the petals fall, the hip begins to grow reddish. When it is bright red, the time for harvesting this powerhouse of vitamin C has arrived. The wild rose yields a hip that is richer in vitamin C than the cultivated rose. Rose hips can be used either fresh or dried (carefully dried hips should be a definite red color) to make tea, jam, syrup, and even soup. The hips do, however, lose a healthy percentage of their vitamin C in the drying.

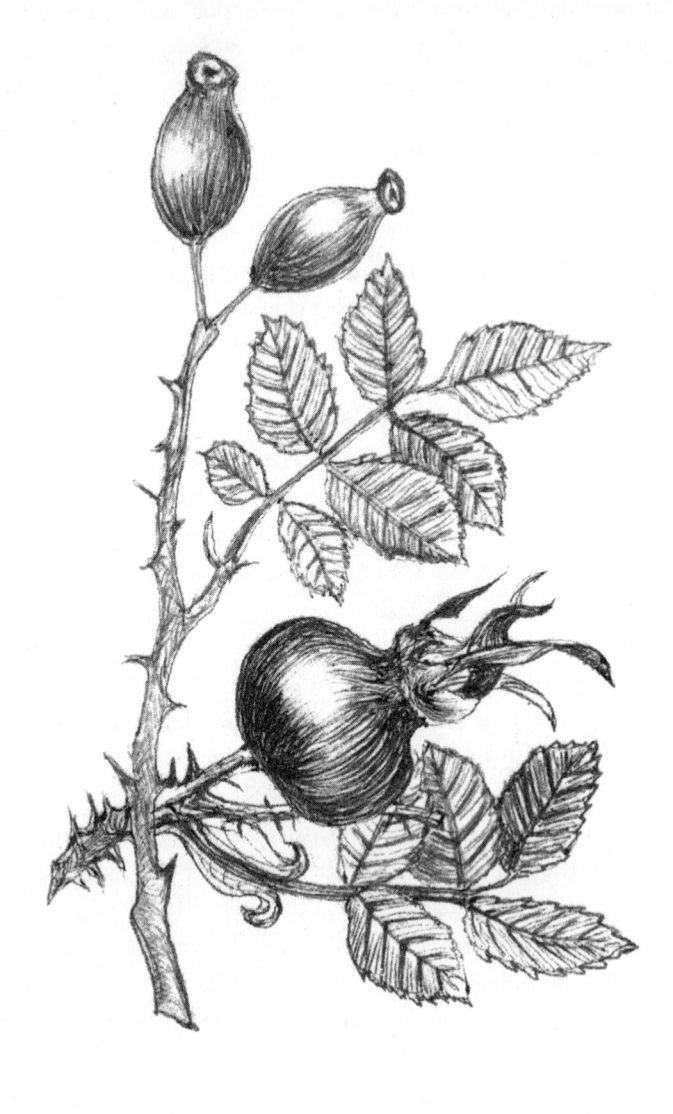

**ROSE HIPS—
TEA ROSE**
approximately ⅔ size

To make rose hip tea, place 2 heaping teaspoons dried hips in a warmed teapot. Add 2 cups boiling water. Cover and steep for 20 minutes. Enjoy it plain; or add honey and lemon. Because of its high vitamin C content, it is excellent by the potful for the cold sufferer. Good for children, and in a bottle for infants. It is also said to be helpful to kidney and gallbladder functions. And its rose color is a joy to behold.

The rose hip is not the only part of the rose that is edible. Rose petals will add delicate flavor to everything from conserves and omelets to cakes and candies. Rose water, which is distilled from rose petals, is widely used in cooking in the Middle East. Rose water is also a cosmetic item, as is the essential oil of the petals, used to soften and gently scent the skin. Attar of roses is the most sought after (and most expensive) of essences—it takes 4,000 pounds of handpicked Rosa damascena petals to yield but 1 pound of perfume essence.

ROSE HIP POWDER   Powdered dried rose hips can be added to soups, breads, cookies, and candies. Blended together with ice water, honey, and lemon, rose hip powder will give you a refreshing summer drink. The powder is rich in vitamin C and has the gentle, pleasant taste of rose hips.

ROSEMARY   In its natural Mediterranean habitat, this savory shrublike herb grows to heights of 6 feet. Its small pointed leaves yield a flavor that no cook should ignore. Rosemary is a natural companion to lamb, and sprigs can be inserted through slits into a roast or used in marinades. All other meats and fish accept rosemary's flavor gladly, but use it with a sparing hand until you are familiar with its potency.

Medicinally, rosemary has been appreciated for centuries as an antiseptic and was used as a strewing herb to scent and disinfect sick rooms. Rosemary tea is useful for nervous conditions, headaches, and digestion and is an effective mouthwash. It stimulates growth of hair when applied externally as a rinse, as well as when it is taken internally as tea. Rosemary oil is also good for the hair; it combats dandruff and makes hair more manageable and easier to comb.

As you grind dried rosemary in your mortar or chop it fresh for Italian focaccia, you may recall (rosemary *is* for remembrance) that this herb is heavy with legends. It is said to have reached the height of Jesus Christ and at his death to have stopped growing upward and started spreading outward. The Virgin Mary purportedly threw her blue cloak over a rosemary bush, turning its white flowers to blue. The herb is said to stimulate brain activity and Greek students wore garlands of rosemary when going into examinations. It has long been a symbol of fidelity and in eighteenth-century England was carried in bouquets by brides and baked in wedding cakes. The smell of rosemary wood is said to preserve youth. The British claimed that the herb would not flourish unless the mistress became master of her household—sending wary husbands out in dark of night to uproot flourishing rosemary bushes!

FOCACCIA

1 tablespoon dried yeast

1 cup lukewarm water

1 teaspoon honey

1 teaspoon salt

2 teaspoons dried rosemary (or 1½ teaspoons chopped fresh rosemary)

7 tablespoons olive oil

1½ cups unbleached white flour

1½ cups whole wheat flour

1 teaspoon coarse salt (optional)

- Dissolve yeast in lukewarm water and let stand until it begins to foam (about 5 minutes). Add honey, salt, rosemary, and 1 tablespoon olive oil. Sift in half of the flour and stir well. On a floured board, knead in the remainder of the flour.

- Pour 2 tablespoons oil into a 9-by-13-inch pan or a 13-inch-diameter pizza pan. With floured fingers, press dough into pan in an even layer. Poke holes with fingers at random, every 2 inches or so, in dough. Pour remaining 4 tablespoons oil over dough and spread evenly with fingers. Sprinkle lightly with coarse salt if desired.

- Bake in a 400-degree oven for 25 minutes or until well browned. Cut in rectangles or pie-shaped pieces and serve warm with soup. Delicious, too, warmed over for a second using.

- Serves four to six.

ROYAL JELLY   Royal jelly is a pale, creamy, sweet substance that is produced by the worker bees to feed the queen bee. The fact that a worker bee lives only a few months while the queen bee can live for three years has aroused much interest in royal jelly. Health food speculators have pounced on it as a miracle substance, a veritable fountain of youth, and there is no doubt that exaggerated claims have been made. However, analysis shows that royal jelly is extremely rich in B vitamins, particularly pantothenic acid, which is known to alleviate many of the diseases associated with aging—such as ulcers, graying hair, heart damage, etc. Royal jelly should be eaten fresh and kept refrigerated.

This expensive item is sometimes added to cosmetics, for which fantastic and rather dubious claims are often made.

RUE   This bitter herb was often used in medieval Europe to flavor salads and omelets. Today it is still used as an herb tea to soothe headaches, nerves, menstrual pains, and infant colic. Brew 1 teaspoon dried leaves in 2 cups boiling water.

RYE FLAKES   Crushed rye grain makes a hearty breakfast cereal, a welcome variation on the usual oatmeal theme. Use 2 cups water or milk to ½ cup rye flakes and simmer for 30 minutes. Serve lightly salted with butter and honey. See also *Rye Grain*.

RYE FLOUR   Rye flour is low in gluten, and it takes an experienced bread maker to turn out a good loaf of pure rye bread. When rye flour is combined with wheat flour, however, it takes no special talent to concoct delicious and buoyant rye bread.

The finest rye flour is organically grown, and stone ground from whole non-degermed grain. See also *Rye Grain*.

PUMPERNICKEL BREAD

        1 tablespoon dried yeast
        1½ cups lukewarm water
        1 tablespoon salt
        ½ cup molasses
        2½ teaspoons caraway seeds
        2 tablespoons vegetable oil
        2 cups rye flour (or meal)
        4 cups unbleached white flour (or whole wheat flour)
        1 tablespoon cornmeal

- Dissolve yeast in lukewarm water. When it foams, add salt, molasses, caraway seeds, oil, and rye flour. Stir very well. Add 2 cups wheat flour and stir in vigorously. Empty onto floured board, and knead in remainder of flour. In oiled bowl let rise in a warm spot until double in bulk.
- Punch down and shape into 2 round balls (or a number of small ones, if rolls are desired). Place on an oiled baking sheet dusted with cornmeal and let rise for 45 minutes.
- Bake in a 450-degree oven for 10 minutes, then lower heat to 350 degrees and continue baking for 30 minutes or until hollow-sounding when tapped. For

rolls, bake for only 20 minutes after lowering heat to 350 degrees.

꙳ Makes 2 round loaves or two dozen rolls.

RYE GRAIN   Rye grain is grown in northern regions where wheat cannot subsist. Its distinctive somewhat sour taste is found in North Country cuisines— in Scandinavia, Germany, and Russia.

Rye is rich in minerals and B vitamins, particularly in potassium and riboflavin. Rye grain can be used as a long-cooking cereal, or it can be ground (if you have a small grain mill) to make meal and flour. It is very useful to those who are allergic to wheat.

A poisonous fungus known as ergot, supposedly the cause of the historical hallucinations that plagued young women during the Salem witch trials, can sometimes infest rye. Ergot contamination, though not uncommon in medieval times, is rare nowadays, as rye grains are treated with pesticides to eliminate any chances of ergot contamination. For this reason, it is important to buy organic rye products that have been protected from ergot via careful and meticulous farming techniques as opposed to poisonous chemicals.

RYE GRITS   These cracked rye grains can be used for cereal or as a main-course replacement for rice or potatoes. They require slightly longer cooking than most other grain grits—about 45 minutes. Use about 3 cups liquid to 1 cup rye grits. See also *Rye Grain.*

RYE MEAL   Coarsely ground rye meal will give the crunchy texture that is characteristic of some types of bread. Use it as you would rye flour. This unleavened rye-meal loaf is ideal for canapés. See also *Rye Grain.*

ROGGEN BROT (UNLEAVENED RYE BREAD)

1³/₄ cups boiling water

1 teaspoon salt

1 tablespoon honey

1 tablespoon pressed vegetable oil

4 tablespoons bran (or wheat germ)

¹/₂ cup wheat grits

2 cups rye meal

꙳ Mix together all ingredients in a large mixing bowl. Cover with a plate or towel and let stand overnight.

- The next day, press the mixture firmly into an oiled loaf pan (or 2 smaller loaf pans). Cover pan *very tightly* with aluminum foil. Place a pan of hot water in a 200-degree oven. Put bread in oven and bake for 4 hours.
- Slice very thin. Perfect for canapés and open-face sandwiches. Keep *roggen brot* refrigerated, tightly wrapped in aluminum foil.

S

SAFFLOWER OIL The safflower plant is known as bastard saffron, and for centuries was used primarily as a scarlet dye for silk and for cosmetic rouge. In its native habitat—India, China, the East Indies—its seed was also pressed to yield an oil that served locally for cooking and for lamp fuel.

Chemical analysis has shown that safflower oil is one of the most unsaturated vegetable oils in existence, a fact that has made it extremely popular in cholesterol-conscious North America. Take care, however, to use safflower oil that has been refined as little as possible. The refinement process employed by the large commercial processors destroys the lecithin content of the oil, without which safflower is of little use as a cholesterol reducer. Safflower oil is light and bland, which makes it a good all-purpose oil for kitchen use.

SAFFRON It takes the handpicked stigmas of 4,300 saffron flowers to make 1 ounce of saffron—which explains the high price of this exotic spice. Saffron comes from a small crocus (*Crocus sativus*) that was first cultivated many centuries ago in Persia and Kashmir.

Saffron has long been valued as a dye and medicine, as well as a culinary spice. The orange-yellow tones of its dyestuff have held sacred positions in widespread areas of the world. There are the saffron robes of the Buddhist monks, the saffron cloaks once worn by Irish kings, and the saffron shirts allotted to noblemen of the Hebrides through the seventeenth century. In the time of Henry VIII of England, ladies of the court took to dying their hair with saffron; they soon found a less expensive method, however—marigolds. The temptation to adulterate saffron has always been strong. In the fifteenth century regular saffron inspections were held in Nuremberg, and culprits were burned at the stake or buried alive—with their impure saffron.

Medicinally, tea made of saffron is a mild stimulant and antispasmodic. But its price is such that one would just as soon find a remedy elsewhere.

In realms culinary, Italian risotto con fungi, Spanish *arroz con pollo*, and French *bouillabaisse* all demand the slightly bitter taste and flamboyant color of saffron. And the highest quality saffron is imported from these countries. Saffron is available powdered or whole, in thin dried threads. Whole saffron should be well crushed in a mortar before using. Remember that a pinch of this spice will carry you a long way.

🌾 FISH FILLETS IN SAFFRON-NUT SAUCE

COURT BOUILLON:
>   5 cups water
>   1 small bay leaf
>   ½ cup sliced carrots
>   1 medium-size onion, halved and stuck with 4 cloves
>   2–3 sprigs parsley
>
>   2 pounds fish fillets, preferably a firm white fish
>   1 medium-size onion, chopped
>   ¾ cup fresh parsley, chopped
>   2 cloves garlic, chopped
>   ¾ cup pecans
>   ¼ teaspoon saffron
>   1 teaspoon salt
>   ⅛ teaspoon freshly ground black pepper
>   2 teaspoons unbleached white flour, if necessary
>   Juice from ½ lemon

- Place all the ingredients for the court bouillon in a fish poacher or pot large enough to hold the fillets, cover and simmer for 30 minutes.
- Add fish, adjust heat as low as possible (the fish should just barely simmer), cover tightly, and cook about 8–12 minutes, or until the fish flakes when tested with a fork. Lift out fish very carefully so as not to break it, and place it on a warm platter in a warm spot.
- While the court bouillon is cooking, prepare onions, parsley, and garlic, and place in a blender along with the pecans, saffron, salt, and pepper. When the fish has been removed from the pot, strain 2 cups court bouillon into the blender, and blend for about 4 minutes, until the sauce is very smooth.
- Pour the sauce into a saucepan and heat but do not boil. If necessary, thicken

with 2 tablespoons unbleached white flour. Add the lemon juice and pour the
hot sauce over the fish.

Serves four.

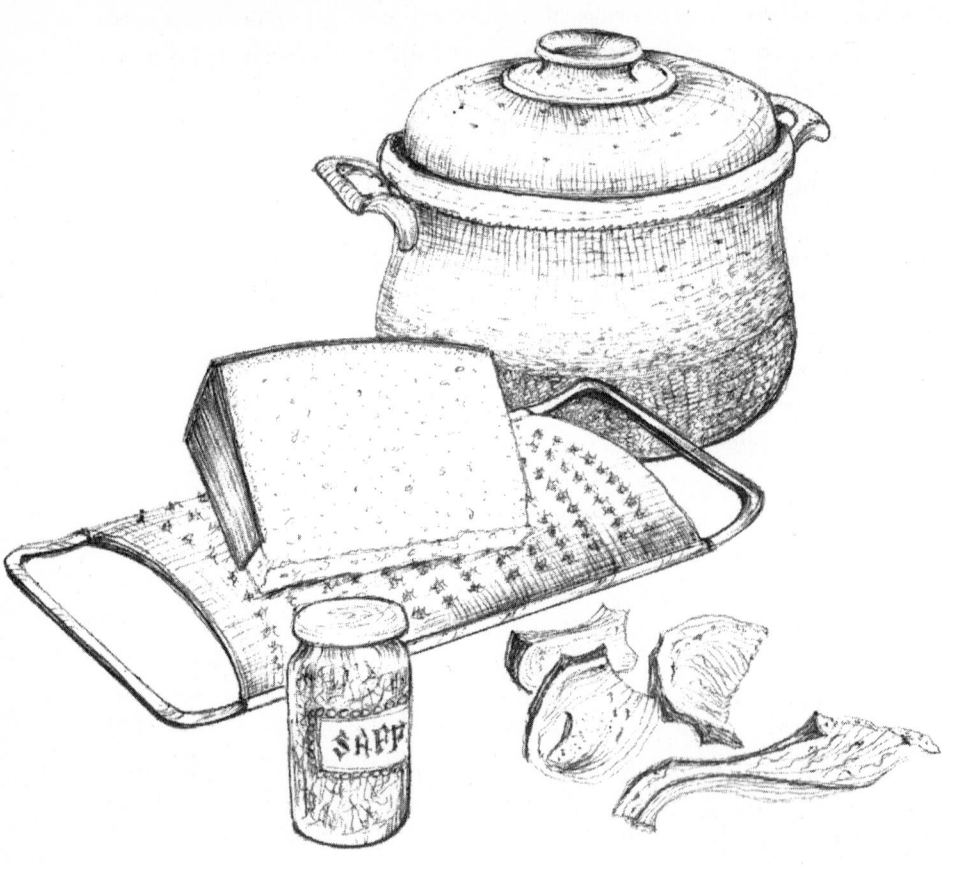

SAGE   How could a man die if he had sage in his garden? asked the ancients.
This herb was once relied upon to cure all manner of ills—from colds to worms,
from excessive sexual desire to sexual debility, from nerves to dandruff and gray
hair. And surely there was some basis in fact for these claims, for sage comes
directly from the Latin word *salvere*, to save. But sage's position in medical cir-
cles is not what it used to be, and no doubt we are the losers.

Sage has a pungent flavor that must be handled carefully in the kitchen. When
sage is not properly dried, it assumes a strong and undesirable musty flavor; try to
use fresh sage or well-treated freshly dried sage. This herb is often added to boost

the flavor of bland meats such as chicken and veal and is a standard ingredient in all types of stuffings. It has long served in the preparation of rich meats and fish, such as sausage, pork, duck, and cod, and sage is said not only to enhance their flavor but to make them more digestible as well. A cup of sage tea is also a pleasant way to aid digestion; pour boiling water over 2 teaspoons fresh chopped sage or 1 tablespoon dried sage and steep for 20 minutes, add honey and lemon.

CHICKEN "BIRDS"

1½ pounds chicken breasts
6 fresh sage leaves (or 2 tablespoons ground sage)
½ cup Parmesan cheese, grated
Freshly ground black pepper
½ cup unbleached white flour
½ teaspoon salt
1½ tablespoons butter
1½ tablespoons olive oil
½ cup dry white wine (or dry vermouth)
Toothpicks

- Have chicken breasts thinly sliced and pounded thinner. Cut into pieces approximately 2 by 3 inches. At end of each piece place one-quarter of a fresh sage leaf or a pinch of dried sage, a generous pinch of Parmesan cheese, and a few grains of freshly ground pepper. Roll up the chicken breast and fasten with a toothpick. When this is finished you should have about 30 small "birds." Combine the flour and salt in a small bowl. Roll the chicken in the salted flour.
- In a large frying pan melt the butter and oil over medium heat. Add the chicken and sauté, turning to brown each side. This should take about 5 minutes. Then add the wine, stir gently with a wooden spoon until the wine evaporates a little and a slightly thick sauce begins to form. Cover the pan for 1 minute.
- Uncover and remove chicken to a warm serving platter ringed with polenta or brown rice. Stir sauce, scraping scraps from the bottom of the pan and incorporating them into the sauce; add more wine if necessary. Spoon sauce over the chicken.
- Serves four.

SAINT JOHN'S BREAD　　See *Carob Pod.*

SALT, SEA   Sea salt is produced by the evaporation of seawater. It contains an abundance of trace minerals (iodine in particular) that make it superior to the pure chemical sodium chloride of land-mined salt. The sea salt richest in minerals is gray in color; next in health value comes the carefully washed white sea salt for table use; third is the white sea salt that has been treated with additives to make it noncaking and free flowing.

Rock salt is found in land deposits where millions of years ago there were probably living seawaters. The passage of time has removed all trace minerals and left the pure chemical, sodium chloride, which many nutritional authorities consider detrimental to health. Commercially processed salt also contains a number of additives that are undesirable in themselves to make it more "manageable"—read labels with care. Detrimental or not, most people in this country use this chemical in abundance. Therefore, some nutritionists recommend purchasing iodized salt, particularly in goiter-prone areas. (Goiter is an iodine-deficiency disease.) A more natural way to supply oneself with iodine, however, is to eat fish, kelp, Swiss chard, turnip and mustard greens, summer squash, watermelon, cucumber, spinach, asparagus, and kale—all rich in iodine—and if you are a vegetable gardener, fertilize your plot with fish emulsion or seaweed.

Although we hear much talk nowadays of the harmful effects of salt, remember that salt is essential to human life and has been valued highly in times gone by—and still is today, in inland Africa and South America. To Homer, salt was "divine," and Plato labeled it a "substance dear to the gods." In many countries it has been valued as money. And we still speak of people being the "salt of the earth," and of those who are "not worth their salt."

Today, however, salt is often misused. It is widely employed commercially to disguise the taste of chemical preservatives and of inferior products. And in the kitchen it too often provides a cover for the blandness of improperly cooked food. Try eating a lightly steamed string bean and see how little salt—if any—it really needs. Salt is absolutely necessary to the life of man. But in these days when baby food, frozen vegetables, canned goods, baking soda and powder, prepared meats, soda pop, nuts, many snacks, and even drugs are loaded with chemical salt, one's concern should certainly be with getting too much, not too little. Use it sparingly, and when you do, use sea salt. Purchase a salt grinder and some fleur de sel from Normandy, France, and you will savor a healthful salt at its best.

SARSAPARILLA TEA   Sarsaparilla tea is made from the dried root of a vine (*Smilax officinalis*) native to tropical America. It was introduced into Europe in the sixteenth century by returning Spaniards and began to be widely used as a cure for venereal and skin diseases. Recent chemical analyses have shown that sarsaparilla contains a number of valuable hormones that lend credence to the old tales of its power over waning virility, loss of hair, psoriasis, and syphilis.

In Asia there is a root (*Smilax china*) with similar attributes, known to us as China root. American sarsaparilla (*Aralia nudicaulis*) is another of the substitutes for Smilax sarsaparilla.

SASSAFRAS TEA   This aromatic tea is made from the bark of the roots of the native American sassafras tree. The chopped whole smaller roots may be used if you don't care for the bark-stripping exercise, but avoid thick pieces of larger roots—they lack flavor. Boil the chopped bark or small roots until the liquid is a reddish-amber tint and a heady aroma wafts up; do not make it too strong or it will become bitter. The same bark can be reused several times before losing its potency.

Sassafras tea was used by the American Indians, who introduced it to the early colonists. It was prized as a blood-purifying tonic and gave relief from all manner of ills—rheumatism, colic, bladder ailments, and such.

If summer flies bother your bowl of fresh fruit, place a few pieces of sassafras root in the bowl and the flies will vanish—so they say. Ground sassafras leaves are used in the filé powder that seasons and thickens the Creole gumbos of New Orleans.

SAVORY   Savory is known as the bean herb, for it not only augments the flavor of dried beans but also aids in their digestion and helps to prevent flatulence. Savory's slight peppery flavor, fresh or dried, is also excellent in salads, soups, sausage, fish, and poultry. Crush savory leaves on a bee sting to reduce swelling and pain. Chew the leaves for sweetened breath and brew them as tea for relief of indigestion and fever.

SEITAN   Seitan, otherwise known as "wheat-meat," is so distinctly meatlike in consistency that some vegetarians avoid it simply because it gives them the willies. Seitan is made from high gluten flour that has been excessively kneaded and rinsed until the wheat starch has been removed, and then simmered, and flavored or marinated. Great in stir-fries, casseroles, stews, and Asian noodle dishes, seitan is less likely to fall apart than tofu and works well as a high-protein additive to many recipes.

SEMOLINA   Semolina is coarsely ground durum wheat. Widely used in Italian and Middle Eastern cookery, it is now widely available in the United States.

Couscous, a North African semolina product, can be substituted in recipes calling for semolina, although the texture of the dish will not be as fine because of the more granular consistency of couscous.

❦ SEMOLINA GNOCCHI

4 cups milk
$\frac{1}{2}$ teaspoon salt
8 tablespoons (1 stick) butter
1 cup semolina
$\frac{3}{4}$ cup Parmesan cheese, grated

- Put milk in saucepan with salt and 2 teaspoons butter; bring to scalding point. Sprinkle in semolina very slowly, stirring with a wire whisk to prevent lumping. Cover and cook over very low heat for 30 minutes. Stir in 1 tablespoon Parmesan cheese.

- Dampen a wooden board or cookie sheet and spread out the semolina in a $\frac{1}{2}$-inch-thick rectangle. Square the edges and smooth the top with a spatula and cool for 15 minutes. Cut into squares about $1\frac{1}{2}$ by $1\frac{1}{2}$ inches.

- Preheat oven to 375 degrees.

- Melt remaining butter and pour one-third of it into a pan large enough to hold gnocchi spaced out so that they don't quite touch each other; individual oval ovenproof serving dishes work well for this also. Place gnocchi in pan. Sprinkle them with the Parmesan cheese and pour over the remainder of the melted butter. Bake for 30 minutes until browned well and bubbling.

- Serves four.

SESAME SEED   These tiny seeds are grown principally in East Asia and to some extent in Africa. African slaves first introduced the sesame seed to America, and in the Southern states it came to be known by its African name, *benne*. These seeds are extremely high in calcium, potassium, iron, phosphorus, and unsaturated oil and contain a good amount of protein. Always purchase the unhulled variety, for many of these nutrients reside in the hull. Organic, unhulled sesame seeds should not all be the same color—they range from very pale brown to tan—uniformity means they have been bleached or hulled.

Sesame seeds are usually toasted before using. This is easy: Place them in a heavy skillet over medium-high heat and stir until they are lightly browned. They are used whole or ground into meal (in a blender or with a mortar and pestle) in cereal and rice dishes, as breading for meats and vegetables, and in and on top of bread and cookies. Whole toasted sesame seeds are a welcome addition to French and Italian salad dressing. Ground sesame seeds are the main constituent of that most delicious Middle Eastern confection, halvah. Raw unhulled sesame seeds can be grown into tasty sprouts.

SESAME SEED COOKIES

12 tablespoons (1½ sticks) butter
1 cup honey
½ cup sesame seeds
1 egg, beaten
1 teaspoon vanilla extract
1 cup plus 3 tablespoons unbleached white flour
¼ teaspoon salt

- Preheat oven to 350 degrees. Oil baking sheets.
- Cream butter and honey well. Roast the sesame seeds lightly in a heavy skillet (see above). Add egg, sesame seeds, and vanilla to the creamed mixture. Add flour and salt and blend well.
- Spoon by the teaspoonful onto an oiled baking sheet, spacing the batter well for it tends to spread out. Bake for 4–5 minutes.
- Makes about 50 cookies.

BAKED CHICKEN WITH SESAME SEEDS

¾ cup toasted sesame seeds
¼ cup unbleached white flour
1 teaspoon paprika
½ teaspoon salt
½ teaspoon pepper
1 (3-pound) chicken, cut in pieces
2 tablespoons pressed vegetable oil

- Preheat oven to 350 degrees.
- Mix together dry ingredients. Dip chicken in vegetable oil and then into sesame mixture. Place chicken, bone side up, in an oiled baking dish. Bake 15 minutes, then turn and bake 45 minutes more.
- Serves four.

SESAME SEED OIL   The oil pressed from the sesame seed is light, mild, and healthfully unsaturated. It is fine for salads as well as cooking and is widely used in Indian cuisine. Sesame oil is also used in making soaps, shampoos, and skin lotions.

SESAME SEED OIL, ROASTED   Roasted sesame seed oil is pressed from the roasted sesame seed, and just as healthfully unsaturated as its unsaturated counterpart. It is dark in color and has a rather strong flavor. It can be used for cooking and salads.

SESAME TAHINI   Made from creamed sesame seeds, this delicious spread is found in health food and Middle Eastern stores. It can be used alone as a sauce or spread, or mixed with miso, hummus, honey, peanut butter, or yogurt to make dips and sandwich fillings. See also *Sesame Seed*.

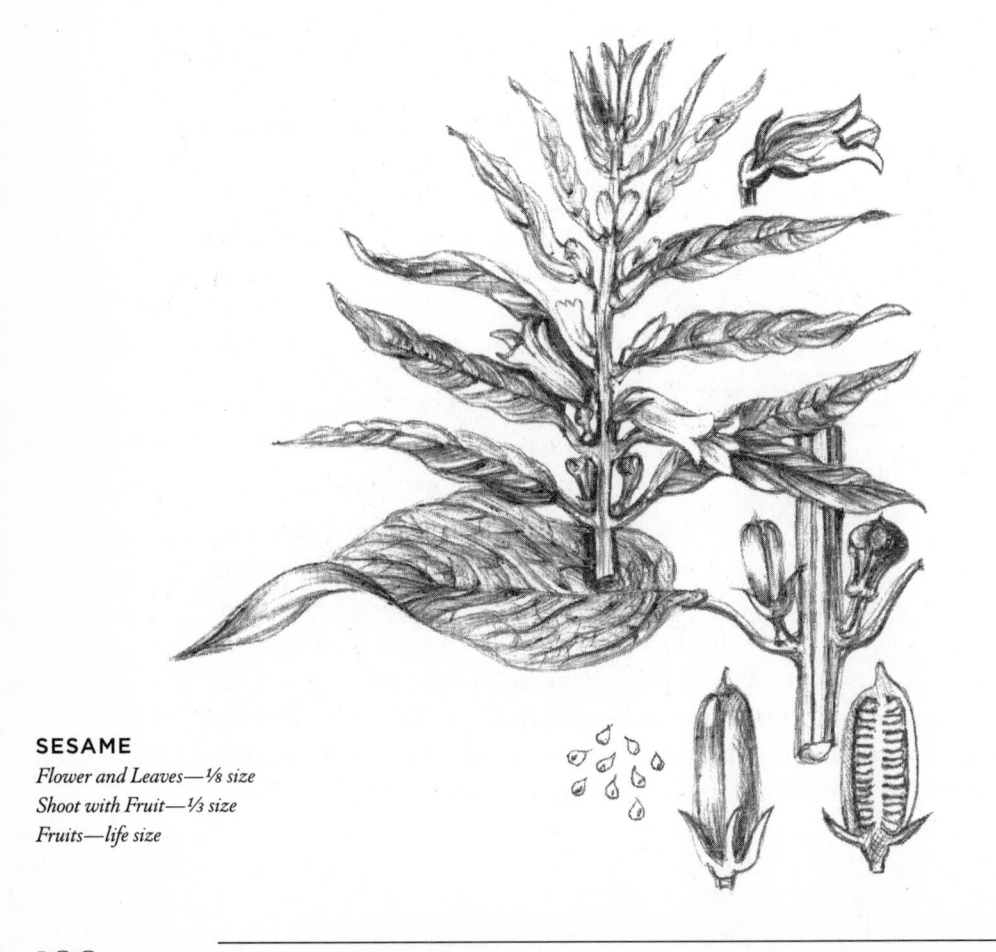

SESAME
Flower and Leaves—⅛ size
Shoot with Fruit—⅓ size
Fruits—life size

SESAME TAHINI

1 cup sesame seeds, raw

1 tablespoon wheat germ, raw or toasted

6 tablespoons sesame oil (preferably pressed oil)

⅛ teaspoon salt

- Grind sesame seeds and wheat germ to a powder in a blender. Place in a bowl and add the sesame oil and salt and mix well. It should have the consistency of peanut butter. Keep refrigerated in a covered jar.
- Makes about one cup.

SHAVE GRASS   The stems of a botanically ancient plant known as horsetail or pewter grass (it is said to be an efficient pewter cleanser) are used to make shave grass tea. It is a kidney and bladder remedy, aids in dissolving kidney stones, and is useful in treating arthritis pain. Shave grass is available as a tea or tincture.

Horsetail (*Equisetum*) plants in large quantities can cause poisoning in livestock.

SLIPPERY ELM   The slippery elm tree (*Ulmus fulva*) is much smaller than the stately American elm. Its bark is used as a remedy for many complaints. The American Indians taught the early settlers how to chop the bark and brew it as a tea to relieve inflammation of the stomach and intestines, sore throats, diarrhea, and dysentery. The hot or cold tea may be applied as a poultice to soothe boils and burns. The bark can also be ground to a fine powder that is used to make throat lozenges to relieve coughs and sore throats.

SOBA NOODLES   These Japanese noodles are made from a combination of wheat and buckwheat flour (sometimes just buckwheat), and water and are delicious both hot and cold. Often served cold with dipping sauces, soba noodles are available dried; though, like any good noodle, they are superior when fresh. Soba noodles are made by rolling out the dough into a thin square, folding, and then cutting by hand into thin noodles. Soba noodles are considered to be more nutritious then semolina noodles, as they contain the benefits of buckwheat flour and are high in protein.

SOLIDAGO TEA   See *Goldenrod Tea.*

SORGHUM SYRUP   Sorghum is a type of millet native to Africa and now also grown in the southern United States. Its stalks contain large amounts of levulose sugar (as found in certain fruits and in honey, as opposed to the dextrose sugar of sugarcane). Sorghum syrup is made from the juices pressed from the sorghum stalks. It is not as strong in flavor as molasses, or as high in minerals, but may be used interchangeably in recipes that call for it. This syrup makes a delicious topping for cereals, pancakes, and desserts.

SOY FLOUR   Soy flour is a powerhouse of protein. It is very low in starch, inexpensive, and easy to use. No kitchen should be without it. A product of ground dried soybeans, this flour will boost the nutritive content of a wide variety of foods without interfering with taste or texture. Add it by the tablespoon to hot cereals, soups, stews, sauces and gravies, meat patties and loafs, casseroles, pancakes, cookies, and cakes.

In bread baking, soy flour can replace one-fifth of the wheat flour. It not only adds protein, lecithin, and vitamins E and B to the bread but also gives a smoother texture and richer crust. And the lecithin acts as a natural preservative—bread made partly with soy flour stays moist and fresh at least twice as long as plain wheat bread. This legume flour lacks gluten, however, and must always be used in conjunction with wheat flour when making bread.

Soy flour is available toasted or raw. The toasted flour is yellow and adds good color and a slight nutty flavor to foods. The raw flour is bland in taste, white in color, and often used for malting tofu or soy curd. Low-fat soy flour has had 99 percent of the oil removed. It is a high-protein product, useful to those who are dieting. But remember that the "fat" in soy flour consists of valuable vitamin E and lecithin; and because it lacks lecithin, low-fat soy flour does not have any preservative qualities.

ITALIAN-STYLE BREAD

1 tablespoon dry yeast (or 2 ounces compressed)

2 tablespoons honey

2½ cups warm water

2 tablespoons pressed oil

1 tablespoon salt

2 cups whole wheat flour

1½ cups soy flour

3 cups unbleached white flour

1 tablespoon cornmeal

- Mix yeast and honey into the warm water and let stand until yeast begins to foam. Add oil and salt. Sift in about 4 cups of the mixed flours, and stir very well (the more you stir, the lighter the bread will be).
- Empty onto a floured kneading board, and knead in the remainder of the flour, adding more unbleached white flour if necessary. Let the dough rise in a lightly oiled bowl, covered with a towel and set in a warm spot, until it is double in bulk—about 1 hour.
- Put the dough on the floured board again, and knead out all the air bubbles. Shape the dough into 1 very large Italian loaf or 2 smaller ones. Place the loaf or loaves on a baking sheet sprinkled with cornmeal, and let rise for another 45 minutes. Halfway through this last rising, make several ½-inch-deep diagonal slits along the top of the loaf.
- Bake at 350 degrees for about 50 minutes or until the loaf is brown and crusty and sounds hollow when tapped with a finger. This recipe yields 1 enormous or 2 regular-size Italian loaves that are certain to please the most refined tastes.

SOY GRITS   Lightly roasted soybeans are coarsely cracked to make soy grits. The grits are used primarily as a meat substitute or a food extender. Prepare them by adding 2 cups boiling water to 1 cup soy grits. When the water is absorbed, the grits can be mixed into meat loaves, hamburgers, egg dishes, stuffings, and cereals. The grits are bland and do not alter the taste of the food to which they are added. Soaked soy grits can be refrigerated in a covered jar and used as needed.

SOY MILK   In Japan and China, soy milk is sold by street vendors and in cafés, where it can be purchased hot, cold, sweetened, or flavored with soy sauce, onions, and vegetables as a warming spicy soup. Naturally thick and rich in flavor, soy milk is the most cow-milk-like of the milk alternatives. High in protein, B vitamins, and iron, soy milk is also available fortified with calcium, vitamin D, and vitamin B_{12}. Soy milk can be found fresh, in the refrigerator section of health food stores, or boxed and shelved. In either case, the soy milk should be used within 7 to 10 days of opening.

Keep in mind that each individual brand of soy milk has a distinctly different flavor and consistency. Some are sweeter than others, some thicker, some vanilla-flavored, some sweetener-free. As a general rule of thumb, it is best to sample a number of different brands; always be sure only to purchase soy milk made from organic, non-GMO soybeans. Soy milk can be made at home with some effort, involving a blender, a hot pot of cooked soybeans on the stove, and a bit of a mess. In order to simplify the process, some swear by the purchase of a soy milk maker, a pitcher-shaped machine that is said to create richer, tastier, more problem-free homemade soy milk than can be achieved with even the most earnest stovetop/blender techniques. Remember, soy milk is never an acceptable replacement for breast milk or formula for children under one year of age.

SOY MILK POWDER   Soy milk powder is finely milled soy flour. It is an excellent milk substitute for infants who are allergic to cow's milk. It is highly nutritious and may also be used in cooking, in the same manner as dairy milk.

SOY OIL   Crude pressed soy oil is pressed from the soybean and is filtered but unrefined. Dark in color, it has a nutlike flavor and is high in unsaturated fats. It is excellent for use in baking, and the high lecithin content gives preservative qualities to breads, cakes, and cookies. Soy oil cannot, however, be used for sautéing or frying because of its tendency to foam.

Much soy oil is not pressed and crude. It is extracted by chemical solvents, refined, bleached, deodorized, and preserved. Avoid it.

SOY SAUCE   Soy sauce is a fermentation of whole soybeans, water, salt, and *koji* (mold spores). Shoyu soy sauce is mild in taste and contains wheat, while tamari soy sauce is wheat free and has a bold, more overpowering flavor. Unfortunately most soy sauces available on the market do not undergo the care and time-consuming preparation of the quality traditional soy sauce. Many are not aged long enough, and monosodium glutamate may be added to perk up inferior flavor; preservatives and chemicals are also used to speed up the fermentation process. True soy sauce has no need of additives or preservatives; if it develops a spot of mold on top, just skim it off—the soy sauce will taste as good as ever and does not need refrigeration.

Use a dash of soy sauce in soups or with vegetables, cooked grains, and meats. Its savory flavor will lend distinctive taste to your dinner fare. Remember, however, that soy sauce is quite salty in itself, and adjust the salt in your recipes accordingly.

CHINESE BEEF WITH VEGETABLES

1 pound flank steak
¼ pound snow peas
2 cups Chinese cabbage, coarsely chopped
½ cup soybean (or mung) sprouts

1/4 cup fresh ginger, peeled and thinly sliced

2 large tomatoes, peeled, seeded, chopped

2 green bell peppers, seeded and chopped

2 medium zucchini, thinly sliced

1/2 teaspoon honey

3/4 cup broth or water

2 tablespoons soy sauce

1 tablespoon arrowroot

6 tablespoons peanut oil

1 clove garlic, chopped

1 large onion, sliced

1 tablespoon sliced dry ginger

Salt and pepper

- This sumptuous dish cooks very quickly. Therefore be certain to have the ingredients prepared before you start to cook. Slice the flank steak very thinly (this is sometimes easier if the meat is partially frozen). Chop or slice all the vegetables you choose to use, leaving snow peas and mung sprouts whole. In a small bowl mix the honey, broth, soy sauce, and arrowroot. Place all the prepared ingredients near the stove.

- Put 3 tablespoons oil in a wok or large frying pan, and heat until quite hot, but not smoking. Put half of the meat in pan. Toss it around with a wooden spoon for 1 minute, browning both sides. Place on a warm platter. Cook remainder of the meat in the same manner. Place it on the warm platter.

- Add 3 tablespoons oil to the pan along with the garlic, onion, and ginger. Toss a few seconds, then add the rest of the vegetables. Stir and cook for 3–4 minutes— they should retain their crispness. Remove vegetables to the warm platter.

- Pour the soy sauce mixture into the pan, and stir until slightly thickened. Pour the sauce over the meat and vegetables. Sprinkle with salt and ground pepper and serve immediately.

- Serves four.

SOYBEAN The soybean has been the mainstay of Asian cuisine for thousands of years. The Western world was long ignorant of the taste and nutritional delights offered by this versatile bean. Extremely rich in high-quality protein, calcium, and B vitamins, this is the only legume that contains all of the essential amino acids; thus it ranks with meat, fowl, and fish as a prime protein source. One-half cup cooked soybeans is roughly equivalent to ¼ pound meat in grams of protein contained.

The soybean can be used fresh or dried, as milk or tofu, as flour or grits, as oil or sauce, and as sprouts or roasted snacks. The soybean is low in starch, easy to digest, and mild in flavor. It blossoms under a sprinkling of herbs and lends itself to an infinite variety of culinary treatments.

In Japan, green soybeans, or edamame, are commonly served in their pods with a sprinkling of salt. Edamame are most readily available frozen. Simply boil for five minutes, toss with salt, and serve. Edamame make a great, healthy finger-food for children, who often like the taste and enjoy the fun of sucking the soybeans out of the pod.

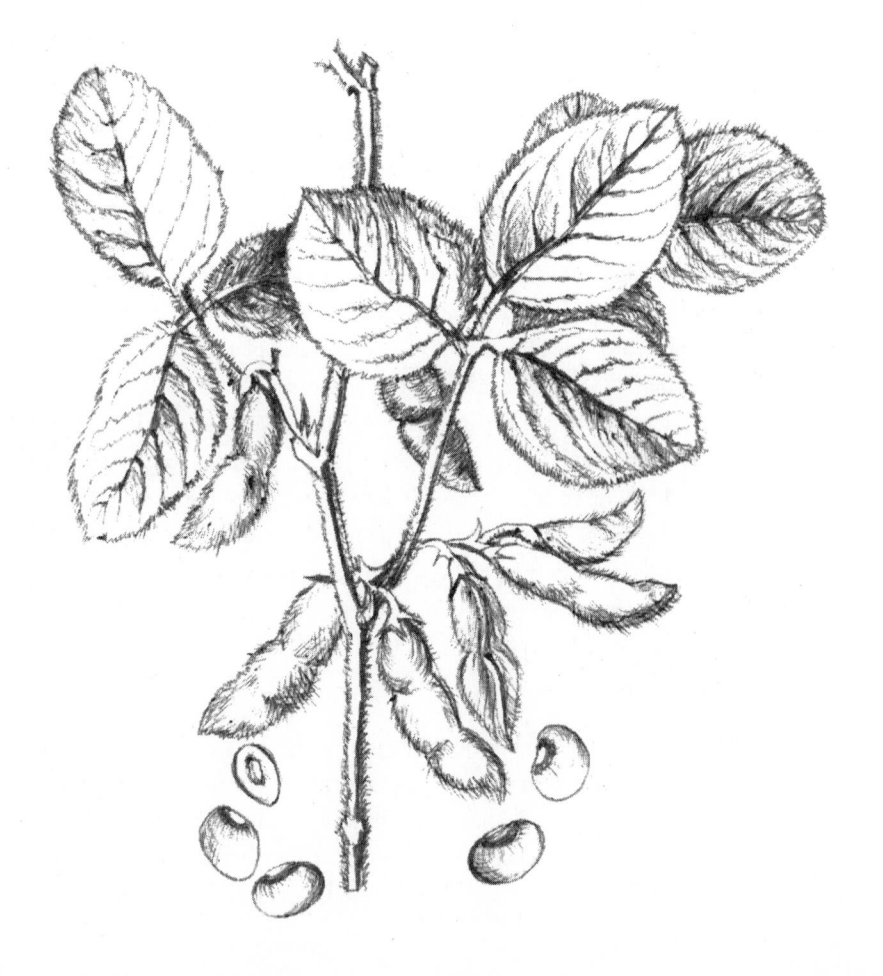

SOYBEAN
Branch and Pods—
approximately ⅔ size
Seeds—life size

❦ SOYBEAN SALAD

Soybeans

½ cup chopped celery

1 medium-size onion, chopped

½ cup chopped fresh parsley

½ teaspoon freshly ground black pepper

½ teaspoon salt

¼ teaspoon dill weed

½ cup mayonnaise (homemade preferred!)

- Wash 2 cups dried soybeans, cover with 1½ quarts water, and soak overnight. If the weather is warm, soak soybeans in refrigerator to avoid fermentation.
- The following morning, put the soybeans and their soaking water in a soup pot, add more water to cover if necessary; add 1 teaspoon salt, bring to boil, skim off foam, then simmer for 2 hours or until tender. Drain and cool the soybeans. Save the cooking water for soups, rice, etc.
- Mix soybeans with the rest of the ingredients. Chill well. Serve as a main course on lettuce, garnished with tomatoes, olives, and cucumber slices. Or put alone in a bowl and use as a side dish.
- Serves four to six.

SOYBEAN, ROASTED Roasted soybeans make a tasty healthy snack food. They contain more protein and are less fattening than their roasted-nut counterparts. However, when buying them prepackaged, examine the label carefully to see that no preservatives have been added. Unfortunately the label will not tell you when the soybeans have been fried in cheap, rancid oil. Really, it's best to roast your own. Here's how.

❦ ROASTED SOYBEANS

1 cup dried soybeans

3 cups water

1 teaspoon salt

- Soak soybeans overnight in water. Refrigerate while soaking if the weather is hot. Add salt and simmer for 1 hour. Drain, keeping leftover water for soup stock, and spread the soybeans shallowly in a baking pan.
- Roast in a 375-degree oven for 45 minutes, stirring every 15 minutes or so. The

soybeans are done when they are lightly browned. Sprinkle with salt while still warm. Serve, or store in a tightly covered jar.

SPEARMINT   Spearmint is the mint most often used in cooking—in the ever-familiar lamb sauce and the Southern mint julep. Spearmint lends itself to a wide variety of dishes: mint-flavored butter adds definite flair to cooked vegetables such as carrots, new potatoes, and beets; and salads take on a Middle Eastern air with the addition of a handful of finely chopped mint. See also *Mint*.

SPELT   Though spelt may seem like a "new" thing to many of us (it was reintroduced into the market in the late 1980s), it is in fact one of the most ancient of grains, dating back as far as 5,000 BC. Unlike wheat, which has been hybridized to increase yield and durability, spelt is higher in fiber, protein, vitamins, and minerals. For those who are gluten-sensitive, spelt is a wonderful alternative, as it is widely tolerated by those who cannot tolerate wheat. Hence the increase in spelt breads and other baked products that are popping up with increased frequency on health food store shelves.

Spelt has a tough husk that makes it more difficult to hull, but has the tremendous benefit of protecting the plant from insects. This makes spelt far easier for farmers to grow without the use of pesticides. Spelt has a rich, nutty flavor and yields dense, moist breads. Try a thick piece of spelt bread, toasted, with a slab of cheese, or for the sweet tooth, organic butter and jam. Chances are neither the taste buds nor stomach will miss that glutenous wheat.

SPICES   Today we take spices quite for granted. But only a few centuries ago these same spices were the gold of the Eastern tropics; Europeans intrigued, fought, and died to obtain them. They were valued not only as seasonings but also as preservatives—an invaluable asset in days when refrigeration was far away.

Spices come from the root, bark, stems, leaves, buds, fruit, or seeds of trees and plants, many of which are native to the tropics. They contain strongly aromatic oils that are fascinating to cook with. Some people maintain, however, that these aromatic oils are an irritant to the kidneys and intestines and should be studiously avoided. But to those who have no such doubts, spices in moderation lend excitement to a vast array of foods. Explore them with a light hand and ready palate!

GARAM MASALA

$\frac{1}{3}$ cup whole cloves

$\frac{3}{4}$ cup cumin seeds

6 (3-inch) lengths of cinnamon stick

$\frac{1}{4}$ cup cardamom pods, dried

$\frac{1}{2}$ cup coriander seeds

$\frac{1}{2}$ cup black peppercorns

Spread all spices on a cookie sheet and roast in a 200-degree oven for 30 minutes, stirring from time to time. Remove from the oven and cool. Peel the cardamom seeds by pushing the pods with your thumb on a table. Then grind all spices in a blender, ½ cup at a time. Or follow Indian tradition and grind them in a mortar.

This recipe will make about 1½ cups and should be stored in a tightly covered jar. It will keep for at least 6 months. Garam masala is used as a spice in many true Indian dishes. Following is a recipe that calls for garam masala.

BEEF KOFTA

1 pound ground beef

1 medium-size onion, finely chopped

$\frac{1}{4}$ teaspoon coriander, powdered

1 tablespoon garam masala

1 clove garlic, finely chopped

$\frac{1}{2}$ teaspoon salt

Mix all ingredients together, and shape into balls the size of small walnuts. Refrigerate while preparing the following:

2 medium-size onions, chopped

2 cloves garlic, chopped

6 tablespoons vegetable oil

2 teaspoons chopped ginger, fresh (or 1 teaspoon powder)

2 teaspoons turmeric

2 teaspoons garam masala

1 teaspoon salt

$1\frac{1}{2}$ teaspoons cinnamon

$\frac{1}{2}$ teaspoon ground clove

$\frac{1}{2}$ cup water

2 cups yogurt

- Sauté onions and garlic in oil. Add ginger, turmeric, garam masala, salt, cinnamon, clove powder. Add water and mix well. Put in the meatballs, and sauté them for about 10 minutes or until browned on all sides. Add yogurt, and stir well. Serve over rice or bulgur.
- Serves four.

SPIRULINA   One of the original green superfoods, spirulina is an algae that is rich in nutrients. Spirulina is high in protein, contains a range of amino acids, and is high in vitamins such as B complex, as well as beta-carotene, iron, calcium, magnesium, manganese, potassium, selenium, zinc, and bioflavonoids. Spirulina is said to be useful in the treatment of allergies and asthma, and has immune-enhancing properties as well as providing sustained energy levels that far surpass the temporary jolt provided by a cup of coffee.

Spirulina is available in tablet, capsule, and powder form. The recommended daily dosage is 3–5 grams. Try mixing spirulina powder in with a smoothie for a nutritional morning treat. A word of caution—spirulina grown in water contaminated by heavy metals can concentrate these toxins. Infectious organisms may also be present and can contaminate the harvested algae. For this reason it is important to find a reputable source of spirulina that has been grown and cared for in a controlled environment. In other words, don't try harvesting your own algae by scraping the surface of the neighbor's fishpond.

SPROUTS   Make a garden of your kitchen! Raise fresh organically grown greens all year round, even if you haven't an inch of earth to call your own, or any sunshine at all. Any seed can be sprouted—alfalfa, mung, soy, lentil, grain, fenugreek, pea, garbanzo, bean—and with the sprout comes a great burst of new energy. Sprouts contain nutrients that do not exist in the seed; they are marvelous sources of vitamins B and C, minerals, and protein.

Growing sprouts is very simple. First make certain to buy seeds that are fresh and untreated with fungicides. Alfalfa is one of the most satisfying seeds to sprout—the taste is mild and delicious; they are nutritious, and beautiful to look at. A mere 3 tablespoons of the tiny seeds will give you 4 cups of sprouts within four days.

There are many methods of sprouting. One of the simplest calls for a quart-size Mason jar with a piece of cheesecloth or nylon mesh stretched over the top. Put 1 tablespoon alfalfa seeds in the jar, cover them with water, and soak overnight. In the morning pour out the water through the mesh covering, rinse the seeds, drain, and set the jar on its side in a dark spot. Two or three times a day, rinse the seeds, drain, and set the jar back on its side in the dark. Within 3 to 4 days the alfalfa sprouts will be about an inch long and will completely fill the quart jar. They are ready for eating. Some people recommend exposing the sprouts to sunlight at this point for a day, to develop chlorophyll content. Store the finished sprouts in a plastic bag in the refrigerator, and start a new batch in the Mason jar. All seeds can be sprouted by following this simple method.

Use sprouts in salads, sandwiches, and blended beverages. Sauté them briefly in pressed oil and season with tamari; or add them at the last minute to soup—keeping in mind that too much heat will destroy their nutritive value and dry them out as well.

CHICKEN SALAD WITH SPROUTS

    4 chicken breasts, skinned and boned
    2 tablespoons olive oil
    3 teaspoons dried dill (or 2 tablespoons fresh)
    3 boiling potatoes, medium size
    3 hard-boiled eggs, sliced
    ½ cup sour dill pickle, chopped
    ½ cup soybean sprouts (or other sprouts)
    1 teaspoon salt
    ⅛ teaspoon freshly ground black pepper
    ¾ cup mayonnaise
    ¾ cup sour cream
    1 tablespoon capers
    1 teaspoon dill weed

Garnish with:

    lettuce
    tomatoes
    watercress

- Preheat oven to 350 degrees. Coat chicken breasts with olive oil, place on baking sheet, and bake 10 minutes on one side; turn, and bake 10 minutes more, until cooked through. Slice breasts into 1×2-inch slices. Chill in the refrigerator.
- Steam potatoes until tender, slice, and refrigerate briefly. Mix together sliced eggs, dill pickles, bean sprouts, salt, pepper, 2 teaspoons dill, chicken, and potatoes in

a bowl. In another bowl, mix the mayonnaise, sour cream, capers, and 1 teaspoon dill. Stir half of this sauce into the chicken mixture.

- ❧ Spoon chicken salad onto a bed of lettuce, garnish with tomato wedges and sprigs of watercress, and pour remainder of sauce over the salad. Serve well chilled as a main course.
- ❧ Serves four.

STAR ANISE   See *Anise Seed.*

STEVIA   Native to Paraguay, this incredibly sweet plant has been used as a sweetener and flavor enhancer for hundreds of years. Virtually calorie free, this sweet plant was once denied access to the United States by the Food and Drug Administration, which apparently preferred more cancerous artificial sweeteners to the completely innocuous and naturally sweet stevia plant. Although it is utilized around the world and favored as a table sweetener in Japan, it was not until 1994 that the FDA would even allow stevia to be marketed in the United States.

Stevia can be used to sweeten any tea or beverage and even in baking, though some experimentation may be necessary, as stevia lacks sugar's ability to feed yeast, add texture, and soften the batter (apparently refined sugar is useful for some things!). But, once accustomed to the unusual sweet taste that stevia imparts, it is well worth the effort, as stevia has virtually none of the dastardly effects of refined sugar. Stevia is available as a powdered extract, a liquid concentrate, and in the form of dried leaves. Stevia plants can be cultivated at home; the fresh leaves can be picked directly from the plant and chewed for a tasty sweet treat. In baking, 1 teaspoon ground powder is equal to 1 cup sugar, and 2 drops liquid is equal to 1 teaspoon of sugar.

SUCANAT   This natural sweetener is made from dried, granulated cane juice. Nothing whatsoever is added, and only the liquid has been removed. Sucanat is composed of small brown granules that have a mild taste, with just a hint of molasses, and may be used one-to-one in replacement of white sugar in recipes. Sucanat is organically grown, so there is never any need to stand in front of the organic and nonorganic options trying to decide how much extra to spend for purity. With sucanat the decision has been made for us!

Not sure if you will like the flavor? Here's a great way to find out. Buy a basket of strawberries in season (organic, of course), place a bowl of sucanat on the table, and dip freshly washed strawberries into the sugar. The sucanat will melt in the mouth in a way that bleached, processed sugar never quite manages.

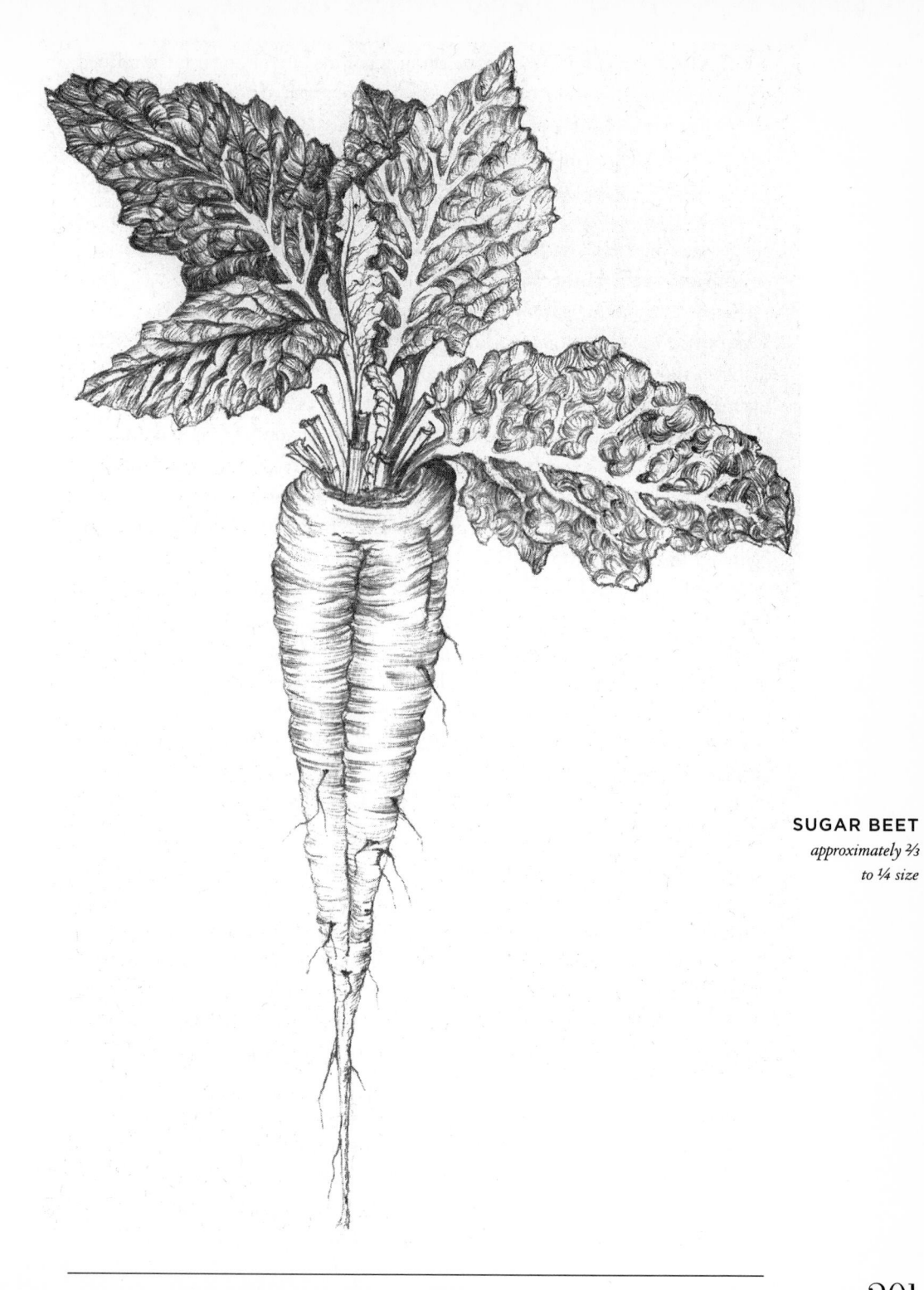

SUGAR BEET
approximately ⅔
to ¼ size

SUGAR, "RAW"   First, a little about sugar in general. Sugar is the refined offspring of the sugarcane or the sugar beet. One hundred years ago the annual per capita consumption of sugar in America was 10 pounds; today it is *100 pounds*. Most of this sneaks into the body very quietly, in processed foods that have sugar added to make them taste "better" (canned vegetables and fruits, peanut butter, dried fruit, fruit juices); and especially in the form of glucose or corn syrup, an utterly tasteless form of sugar that is used as a cheap filler and emulsifier in everything from cheese to catsup.

Refined sugar is an extremely detrimental food. It robs the body of B vitamins and contributes to nervous conditions, tooth decay, pancreas malfunction, acne, diabetes, stomach ulcers—and body tonnage galore. It most certainly is not the harmless high-energy food that sugar manufacturers would have us believe.

And yet the sugarcane itself is regarded as a kind of wonder food. It is said that sugarcane field workers who frequently suck on the fresh cane are notably free from cavities and diseases. (We have as yet to hear of sugar-beet chewing.) Sugarcane contains almost all the nutrients and enzymes necessary to sustain human life; it is rich in vitamin B and minerals.

What happens to all this goodness? It certainly does not end up in the sugar bowl. It goes into the blackstrap molasses that once was dumped as a waste product and is now fortunately recognized as a valuable food. When the molasses is separated from the sugar juices, what is left is true *raw* sugar—sticky dark-colored crystals. This, if one wanted to use the best of sugars, would be the sugar to use. Unfortunately it is not available now in the United States; there are laws preventing the entry of unrefined sugar to these shores.

So the raw sugar is refined and refined and refined until we are left with pure white sucrose. Then to satisfy the health food fans, molasses is poured back over the white sugar—a little bit to give that raw-sugar look; slightly more for the brown-sugar look. It's a put-on! And yet, we buy it! While trying to keep our consumption of this product to the absolute minimum, when the occasion calls for a delicate pastry or sumptuous dessert, we are at least thankful for that little bit of molasses clinging to the sucrose crystals. "Raw" sugar is a step in the right direction, albeit a small one, away from refined sugar and toward more healthful sweeteners such as honey, date sugar, stevia, sucanat, and molasses.

SUN-DRIED TOMATOES   This Italian delicacy is one with such versatility and exquisite results that no kitchen should be without it. Sun-dried tomatoes are available both marinated in oil and herbs or dried. The dried tomatoes can be reconstituted in water and used in a multitude of recipes, from pasta to polenta to pizza. Marinated dried tomatoes can be eaten on crackers with cheese or diced and thrown directly into pasta sauces. High in potassium and iron, sun-dried tomatoes can add zest and depth to almost any dish. During the winter months, when good, fresh organic tomatoes are simply not to be had, try using sun-dried tomatoes instead; while the results will not be the same, the flavor will undoubtedly be richer than anything achievable with those anemic winter tomatoes.

SUNFLOWER SEED The seed of the annual sunflower is too little appreciated in this country. The American Indians once made great use of the entire flower, using the seeds, stalks, and roots for food. In southern Russia the sunflower is widely cultivated for the valuable oil yielded by the seeds and for the seeds themselves. The hulled seeds offer a valuable source of vitamin B, protein, phosphorus, and potassium. Some claim that the seeds gain special energy from the flower's assiduous following of the sun from early morning to sundown.

Hulled sunflower seeds, either raw or lightly roasted, make a delicious snack for children and adults as well. Many of the preroasted varieties of sunflower seeds sold in stores are overcooked (destroying nutrients) in low-quality oil, over-salted, and may have preservatives added. It is best to roast your own—a most speedy and simple process. Remember that the incomplete protein of sunflower seeds is complemented by that of peanuts. Try mixing the two for a snack that is a powerhouse of high-quality protein.

SUNFLOWER SEED–PEANUT ROAST

   1 cup raw hulled sunflower seeds
   3/4 cup raw shelled peanuts
   1 teaspoon soy sauce (optional)
   2 teaspoons pressed vegetable oil
   1 teaspoon salt
   1/2 cup raisins or currants (optional)

- Place a heavy skillet over medium-high heat. Pour in sunflower seeds and peanuts. Stir until a roasted aroma rises and the seeds and nuts start to brown. Add soy sauce if desired. Sprinkle in the oil, stirring to coat everything evenly, then stir in salt.
- Pour into serving bowl, and add raisins or currants.

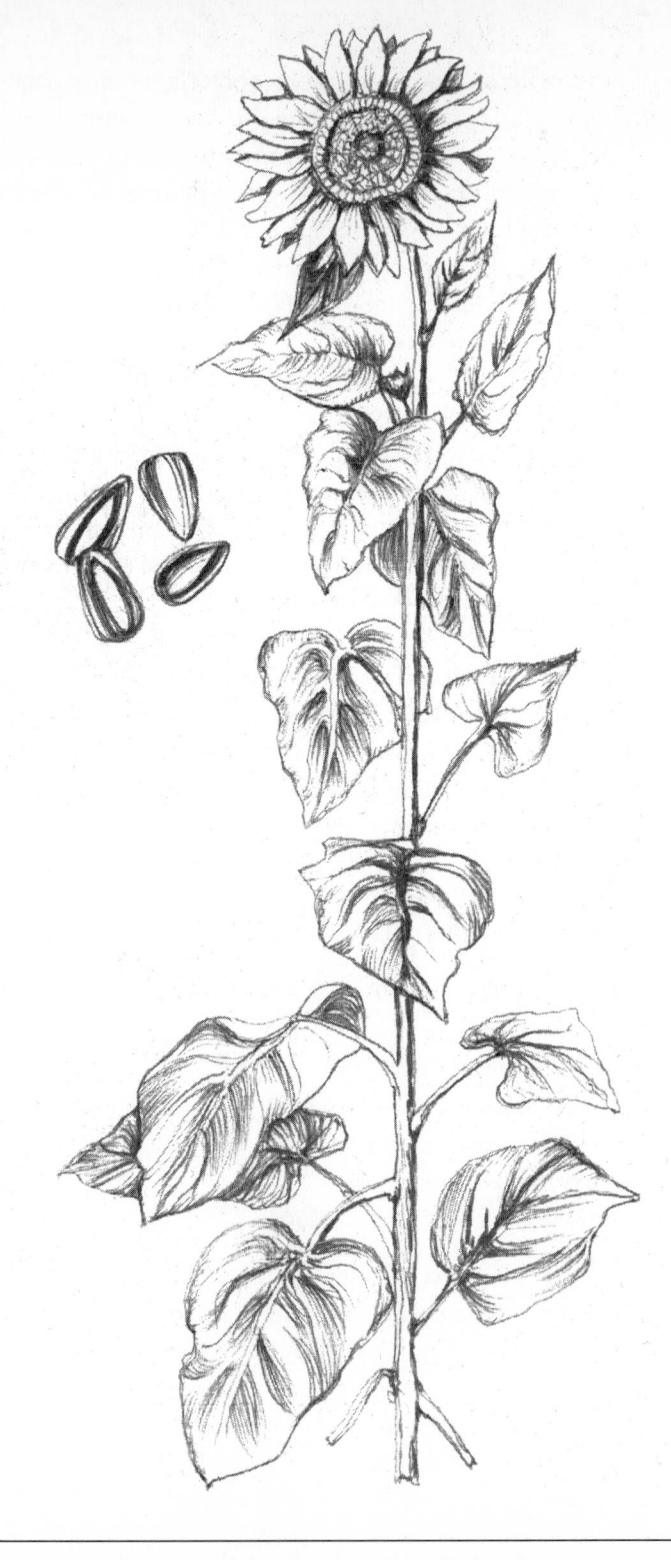

SUNFLOWER

Plant—approximately ⅛ size
Seeds—life size

THE DICTIONARY OF WHOLESOME FOODS

CHEWY SUNFLOWER SEED COOKIES

8 tablespoons (1 stick) soft butter

½ cup honey

2 eggs, beaten

1 teaspoon vanilla extract

1½ teaspoons cinnamon

½ cup whole wheat flour, sifted with bran added back

½ teaspoon salt

1½ cups rolled oats

½ cup raisins

½ cup raw hulled sunflower seeds

½ cup sesame seeds

½ cup shredded unsweetened coconut

- Preheat oven to 325 degrees. Lightly grease cookie sheet.
- Cream butter and honey. Add eggs and vanilla. Then add cinnamon, flour, and salt. When well mixed add oats, raisins, sunflower seeds, sesame seeds, and coconut. Spoon onto cookie sheet. Bake for 12–14 minutes. Cool on rack.
- Makes 50 cookies.

SUNFLOWER SEED MEAL   This meal is made from ground sunflower seeds. Prepare it in a blender (1 cup hulled seeds yields 1G cups meal), or purchase it preground in a health food store; keep it refrigerated. A delicious and healthful addition to soups, cereals, casseroles, breads, and cookies, it cooks quickly and has a mild nutty flavor. When making bread and cookies, one-fifth to one-half of the wheat flour may be replaced with an equal amount of sunflower seed meal. See also Sunflower Seed.

SUNFLOWER DROP BISCUITS

1½ cups whole wheat flour

½ teaspoon salt

2 teaspoons baking powder

½ cup sunflower seed meal

6 tablespoons pressed vegetable oil

2 eggs, lightly beaten

½ cup milk

- Preheat oven to 400 degrees. Lightly oil baking sheet.
- Sift flour, salt, and baking powder into a mixing bowl. Add sunflower seed meal, oil, and eggs. Mix in the milk. Drop by the teaspoonful onto baking sheet and bake for 12 minutes. Serve hot.
- Makes about 2 dozen biscuits.

SUNFLOWER SEED OIL   The oil of the sunflower seed is an excellent source of unsaturated fatty acids. Unsaturated fats are essential to a healthful diet and help keep the blood cholesterol level in line. Be sure to buy pressed sunflower seed oil rather than additive-filled chemically extracted commercial oil. Sunflower seed oil is excellent for salad dressings and cooking.

T

TAMARI See *Soy Sauce*.

TANSY TEA The aromatic leaves of the bright yellow tansy flower (*Tanacetum vulgare*) can be used to make an herbal tea that will bring on delayed menstruation and calm hysteria. Tea made of tansy leaves and seeds is said to expel worms. In medieval times a dish of young leaves cooked with eggs was called a tansy. Tansy tea has a strong taste; in large doses it can be a violent irritant, so brew it mild and use with care.

TAPIOCA Tapioca is a product of the roots of the cassava or manioc plant that is cultivated widely in Africa, South America, and tropical East Asia. Certain varieties of the roots are poisonous when eaten raw but are perfectly safe after cooking.

To make tapioca, the tubers are processed into small round white "pearls"—most commonly used in this country for making puddings. Tapioca consists almost entirely of easily digestible starch and is very low in minerals and protein. It is used mainly in the diets of invalids and young children, and aside from its easy digestibility has little to recommend itself.

TAPIOCA FLOUR Tapioca flour is a farinaceous product of the tropical manioc or cassava root. This fine white flour is an easily digestible starch and is used for thickening broths and gravies. It is not widely available; arrowroot powder is used for the same purposes and is generally easier to obtain in the United States. See also *Tapioca*.

TARRAGON Although tarragon is probably best known as an infusion for vinegar, please don't stop there! This heady and flavorsome herb does wonderful things to fish and is also used to advantage in salads, soups, sauces, and chicken dishes. Traditional French sauces such as béarnaise, hollandaise, and tartar depend on tarragon for their sophisticated flavor. In medieval Europe tarragon was also used as a breath sweetener and soporific.

Unlike most herbs, tarragon is not as pungent dried as fresh, for its essential oils disappear during drying. So use fresh tarragon sparingly and dried tarragon liberally. French tarragon is of higher quality than Russian or "false" tarragon.

Try this delicious and unusual tarragon sauce the next time you serve fish or lamb.

❦ TARRAGON SAUCE

1 pound fresh spinach

1 cup mayonnaise (see recipe in book)

1 cup sour cream

2 tablespoons lemon juice

3 tablespoons dried tarragon (or 1$\frac{1}{2}$ tablespoons fresh)

$\frac{1}{2}$ cup chopped parsley (optional)

$\frac{1}{2}$ teaspoon salt

$\frac{1}{4}$ teaspoon freshly ground black pepper

- Wash spinach well and cook it in the water clinging to its leaves until it is just wilted. Drain well and chop finely. Mix together the other ingredients and stir in the spinach.

- If you use a blender, just blend everything together; the texture may not be as pleasant as when it is chopped by hand, however. Chill and serve with fish or lamb.

- Makes about 3 cups.

❦ GREEN RICE SALAD

2 cups leftover cooked rice

$\frac{3}{4}$ cup cooked green peas

$\frac{3}{4}$ cup tarragon sauce (see above recipe)

- Mix together all three ingredients, and serve chilled on a bed of crisp lettuce or watercress. This is a delicious summer salad.

TEA, HERB   See individual herb teas.

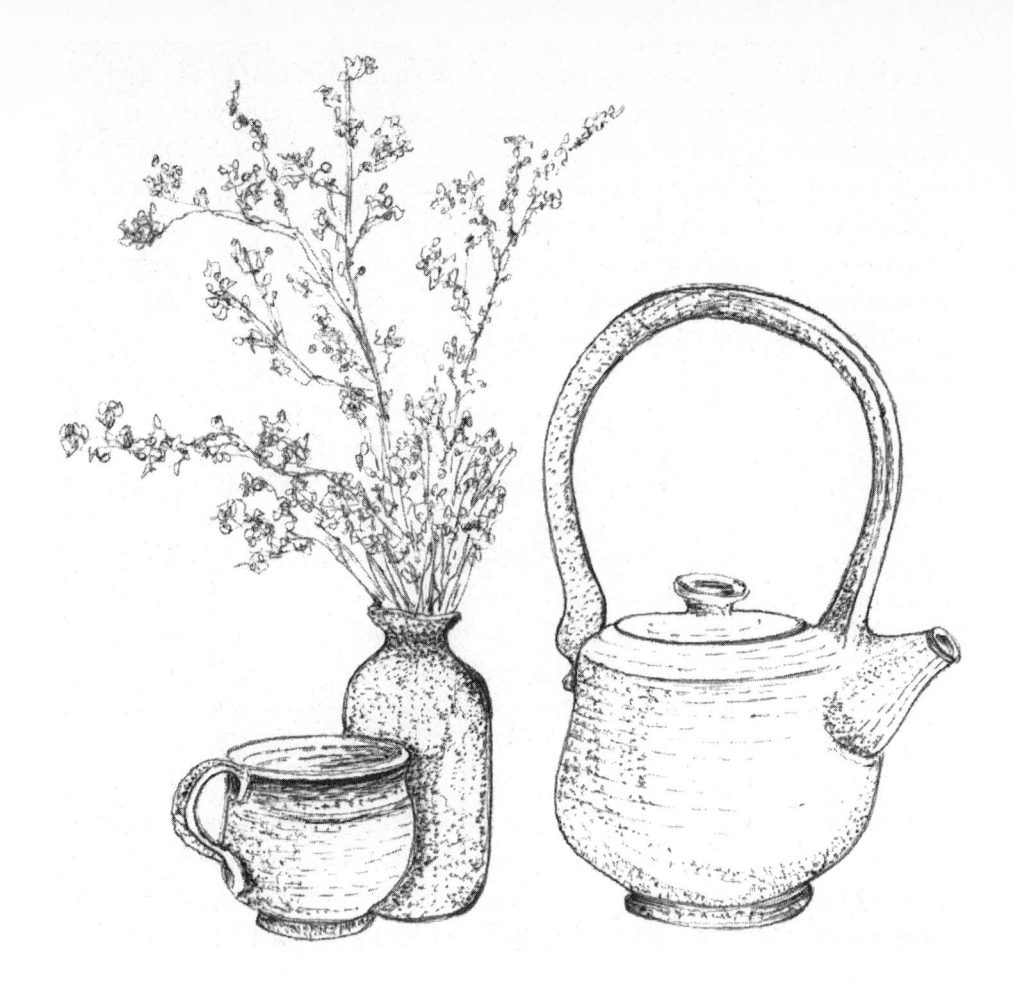

TEA, BLACK The topmost leaves of each branch of the camellia-related tea plant are plucked for making the finest teas This plant flourishes throughout Asia and most of the tropics. The many different varieties of tea all come from the same plant; their differences depend on where the plant is grown, how close to the top of the branch the plucked leaves were, and how the leaves are processed after picking. Black tea leaves are produced by drying, fermenting, and roasting. Green tea leaves are dried and roasted without fermentation. Tea has long been an honored beverage in Asia, where one legend has it that the Buddhist saint Bodhidharma once fell asleep while meditating; he was so distressed at this that he cut off his eyelids so that he might never sleep again. The eyelids fell to the ground, took root, and two tea plants sprang up—whose leaves yielded a brew that could banish sleep.

Tea reached Europe in the seventeenth century and came to America soon after. It was at first regarded with moral and medical trepidation. One essay of the day protested that "men seem to have lost their stature, and women their beauty" due to overindulgence in tea. But the protesters fought a brief and losing battle, for tea was soon overwhelmingly embraced by the Western world.

Nowadays, however, tea is again under attack. Tea contains both tannic acid and caffeine, the same bugbears as coffee. And although 1 cup of tea contains less of these ingredients than coffee, it is still held by some to be an unhealthful stimulant and irritant to the body. Here is a method of brewing that is said to cut down on the tannic acid content of tea: Pour a little boiling water over the tea leaves; let it sit 1 minute; then pour it off, add fresh boiling water, and brew normally. Loose-leaf tea is far preferable to the ubiquitous tea bag. Its flavor is infinitely superior and it does not contain the bleach that is found in many tea bags.

For those who feel that the drawbacks of tea outweigh delights, there are vast numbers of healthful herbal teas to sip and savor.

TEA, GREEN   Rather than being fermented, as black tea leaves, green tea leaves are withered and steamed, or dried after harvest, a process that leaves the tea enzymes active and keeps the antioxidants intact. If consumed on a regular basis, three to four cups a day, green tea is reputed to have anticancer properties, antiallergen activity, to be useful in weight loss, in treating arthritis, and is said to provide mental clarity, which makes green tea particularly useful when fasting. Health benefits aside, green tea is a refreshing, delicious alternative to black tea, as it is low in caffeine and perfect for a subtle pick-me-up at any time of day.

TEA, WHITE   Produced almost entirely in the Fukien province of China, white tea is considered to be even richer in health benefits than green tea, which makes this relative newcomer to the tea lineup well worth steeping. The leaves and buds of the tea plant are neither fermented, withered, nor rolled; they are simply steamed and dried. White tea, therefore, is the least processed of all teas, with the highest remaining antioxidant levels. White tea contains a high proportion of buds, which are harvested before the tea leaves open fully, when the tea buds are still covered in fine white hairs.

While many green teas have what some people consider to be a grassy or bitter flavor, white tea is sweet and mild. The caffeine content is slightly lower than that of green tea and significantly lower than black tea. Thought by many to be the gourmet of green teas, white tea is expensive—but worth the price.

TEFF   This ancient grain is thought to have been domesticated in Ethiopia sometime between 4000 BC and 1000 BC. In Ethiopia, teff is used to make a sourdough flatbread called *enjera*, as well as for porridge and alcoholic drinks. The teff grasses are used in adobe housing and to feed livestock.

Teff grains are minute in size and predominately made up of bran and germ, the most nutritional parts of any grain. High in calcium, iron, barium, thiamin, phosphorous, protein, and fiber, as well as lysine and other amino acids, teff is a gluten-free grain that is truly worth experimenting with. Teff varies in color from light to dark, depending on variety, and has a mildly sweet, nutty flavor that works well in baked goods, soups, and stews. Substitute part of the flour in any recipe with teff flour, or use teff grains to replace part of the nuts and seeds. Teff cooks like rice, but with a 2 cup water to ½ cup teff ratio.

TEMPEH   Looking for a good meat alternative, but tired of tofu? Tempeh could be the perfect solution. Originally from the Indonesian island of Java, tempeh is a staple food in Indonesia. A complete protein food, tempeh is rich in amino acids, riboflavin, magnesium, manganese, and copper, and is reputed to lower cholesterol levels. Tempeh is made by cooking and dehulling soybeans. The beans are then inoculated with a culturing agent, rhizopus, and incubated overnight until a solid cake is formed. Tempeh can be added to any dish, where it will both absorb other flavors and provide a rich, nutty taste of its own.

TEXTURIZED SOY PROTEIN   Available in both granules and chunks, texturized soy protein is made from defatted soy flour that has been compressed. When rehydrated, texturized soy protein has a texture very similar to ground beef or turkey meat. When stored in an airtight container, texturized soy protein can be kept in the cupboard for several months, but once rehydrated, it should be refrigerated and used within a few days.

When used in sauces, soups, and stews, texturized soy protein can be added directly without first being rehydrated. Otherwise, texturized soy protein should be rehydrated by adding roughly 1 cup of water to 1 cup of granules and allowed to simmer for a few minutes. A great source of fiber, texturized soy protein is low in fat and rich in protein. It's a perfect way to add meatlike texture and nutritional enrichment to vegetarian recipes.

THYME   Legend has it that a soup of thyme and beer will cure shyness! Certainly thyme itself is anything but a shy herb. Wherever you plant it, it will spread rapidly; whatever food you add it to, it will tend to dominate. Keep a firm hand on thyme, or it will get the best of you. Its somewhat minty flavor adds good taste to poultry stuffings, salads, and steamed vegetables.

The leaves contain an oil known as thymol, which is antiseptic and used in cough medicines, mouthwashes, and salves. Tea brewed from the dry or fresh leaves has various medicinal effects that have been appreciated for many centuries. It has been used to treat whooping cough, asthma, and throat and lung problems. As a nervine it is said to prevent nightmares. It has been a prime ingredient in herbal pillows, which were once widely used to induce sleep.

CHICKEN LIVER PATÉ

4 medium-size onions, chopped
2 pounds chicken liver (organic)
2 tablespoons vegetable oil
3 hard-boiled eggs, chopped
2 tablespoons cognac (optional)
¼ teaspoon thyme, dried or fresh
Salt and pepper to taste

Sauté onion and chicken liver in vegetable oil until onion is tender and liver is browned. Put in a blender; add eggs, cognac, thyme, salt, and pepper. At medium speed, blend until smooth. If you do not have a blender, chop all ingredients as finely as possible and mash together with a fork.

Press firmly into a bowl and cover carefully with plastic wrap or a thin covering of melted butter. This will keep under refrigeration for about a week; the butter or plastic covering prevents discoloration. Serve with rye crackers as an hors d'oeuvre or luncheon dish.

Makes about 1½ cups.

LAMB SHANKS

Olive oil
4 lamb shanks (4½–5½ pounds total)
Salt and pepper
1 large onion, chopped
4 carrots, chopped
4 parsnips, chopped
4 stalks celery, chopped
1 tablespoon dried rosemary, or 3 tablespoons fresh rosemary
6 bay leaves

6 cloves garlic, chopped

3–4 cups red wine

6 branches fresh thyme, or 2 tablespoons dry

1 lemon, zest and juice

1 orange, zest and juice'

Cornstarch (optional)

🍃 Preheat oven to 350 degrees. Heat oil in large, deep Dutch oven with tight-fit-ting lid. Season lamb with salt and pepper and cook in batches (if necessary), turning with tongs until well browned, about 10–15 minutes for each batch. Remove shanks with tongs to a plate.

🍃 Sauté vegetables, garlic, and herbs for 10 minutes, or until the vegetables are very soft. Add 3 cups of wine, bring to a boil, and simmer for 10–15 minutes. Taste for seasoning. Add salt and pepper to taste. Add shanks to the pot and braise in oven for 90 minutes, turning every 30 minutes. Add lemon and orange juice and braise for another 30 minutes. Add zest. Stir well. If necessary, thicken with a little cornstarch mixed with cold water. Heat through. Garnish with chopped parsley. Serve with couscous.

🍃 You can stop braising at 90 minutes, refrigerate, and reheat the next day for the additional 30 minutes. This improves the flavor and also gives you the oppor-tunity to remove any fat that has accumulated on top of the dish.

🍃 Serves four.

TINCTURE   Considered by many to be the most effective way to assimilate the power of herbs into the body, no health food companion would be complete without mention of the invaluable tincture! Tinctures are made by soaking fresh or dried plant material in a mixture of either alcohol and water, or glycerol. The herbs are put in a jar, covered in the desired liquid, and stored in a dark place for two weeks or so—the jar should be given a good shake every two days—the resulting liquid is then poured off and is ready for use.

Many tinctures are available in glycerol form for children, who often quell at the taste and smell of alcohol-based tinctures. Though these tinctures are sweet to the taste, glycerol is considered to be an inferior way of extracting the power-ful benefits of the herbs, so if a child can be made to choke it down, an alcohol-based tincture is bound to be more effective and powerful. Because the recommended dosage is only 15–45 drops, there is no need to worry about the alcohol content affecting a child. If anything they will develop a powerful aver-sion to the taste!

When mixed with a small amount of water, tinctures are easier to swallow, which can be a helpful tip when dealing with some of the more bitter herbs. Tinctures are an invaluable addition to any medicine cabinet. Useful for both adults and children, they provide a quick and simple way to reap the benefits of natural medicine. Alcohol-based tinctures last for two years or more without deteriorating.

TOFU   Tofu is also known as soybean curd. It is a staple food in China, where it was developed thousands of years ago. Even today, each school of Chinese cookery is said to have its own special way of preparing this delicate food. Tofu is very high in protein (some call it boneless meat) and in vitamin B. It is somewhat bland in flavor, but when well seasoned and combined with other foods, it is a gourmet item. Use it in salads, soups, vegetarian dishes, and desserts. Tofu, much like chicken, absorbs the flavors around it, and is wonderful when marinated before cooking, or added, fresh, to soup broths like the one below.

TOFU-VEGETABLE SOUP

4 cups soup stock (or water)

^{3}/4 cup tofu, diced in 1-inch cubes

1^1/2–2 cups sliced fresh vegetables, assorted

2 teaspoons miso

1^1/2 tablespoons chopped chives (or scallion tops)

Bring soup stock to a boil. Add tofu and vegetables and simmer for 10 minutes or until the vegetables are just tender and still a little crisp. Spoon out a little of the stock and mix it in a small bowl with the miso; add this to the soup, and do not let it boil again. Garnish with chopped chives or scallion tops and ladle out immediately.

This quick and easy soup serves four.

CURRIED TOFU

4 ounces curry paste (generally available in specialty stores)

2 cups coconut milk, unsweetened

1 tablespoon honey

2 tablespoons tamarind sugar

1 tablespoon Thai fish sauce, or if not available, 1^1/2 tablespoons soy sauce

^{3}/4 pound sweet potatoes, peeled, cubed, and parboiled

½ pound string beans, blanched

1 ¼ pounds baked, cubed tofu ("baked" tofu is available at health and specialty food stores)

3 tablespoons chopped Thai basil

2 large onions, chopped and sautéed

- Mix curry paste with coconut milk. Add ½ cup water. Bring to a boil. Add honey, tamarind sugar, fish sauce. Then add potatoes, onions, and beans. Cook until potatoes and beans are done. Add tofu.
- When heated through, serve and garnish with chopped basil. Delicious with either basmati or brown rice.
- Serves four.

TURBINADO   A highly granulated sugar made from the residue left after the sugarcane has been processed to remove the molasses. Real raw sugar, which is produced in the initial stages of white sugar's manufacturing, is not available in the United States, as it is reputed to contain bacteria, molds, or insect parts. Thus, the "raw sugar" we see on the market shelves is most often turbinado, or raw sugar that has been further refined and steam-cleaned to remove such impurities. With a flavor that is much richer than its more refined counterparts, turbinado makes an excellent choice for sweetening teas and coffee and can be used in baking.

TURMERIC   This brilliant orange spice gives curry powder its characteristic golden color and adds a spicy flavor as well. Turmeric is a tuberous root of the ginger family and is native to India. The turmeric root is prepared by washing, peeling, drying, and powdering for use as a dyestuff or as a spice. Turmeric can be added to any curry dish or used alone to lend color and subtle spice to rice, cream sauce, and mayonnaise.

TWIG TEA (KUKICHA)   This Japanese tea is a combination of green tea leaves and its thin white twigs and stems. Lower in caffeine than green tea, kukicha tea has a rich chestnutlike flavor that is well complemented by honey and milk. It's a great alternative for those who wish to avoid the caffeine content of black tea but miss that full-bodied flavor. Twig tea is a perfect late-afternoon blend that is available organic, loose, or in tea bags.

U

UDON NOODLES   Most commonly used in soups, udon noodles are a thick, firm noodle made from wheat, salt, and water. Udon noodles are served cold in the summer months with a dipping sauce. Any sauce will do, but a soy-based sauce called *mentsuyu* is the most common. Try udon noodles with peanut dipping sauce or in a brothy soup. These high-protein noodles are delicious and satisfying.

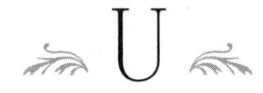

SESAME NOODLES

> 1 pound udon noodles
> 2 tablespoons sesame oil

Sauce:

> 1 tablespoon honey
> ¼ cup tahini (sesame paste)
> ¼ cup soy sauce
> 2 tablespoons wine vinegar
> 1 tablespoon chili pepper oil or ¼ teaspoon crushed red peppers
> 2 cloves garlic, crushed
> 2 teaspoons ginger, grated

Garnish:

> 2 scallions, sliced in 2-inch pieces

- Combine sauce ingredients. Cook noodles according to package directions. Toss with sesame oil. Combine with sauce. Serve hot or cold with sliced scallions on top.
- Serves eight as a side dish.

UMEBOSHI   These are Japanese plums that have been picked before ripening completely, packed in wooden barrels, and then soaked in brine (a strong solution of salt and water used for pickling), and red shiso leaves, which endow the umeboshi with their lovely pink tint. Umeboshi plums are high in protein, calcium, iron, and phosphorous, and are said to aid in the relief of morning sickness and constipation. Umeboshi plums are an alkaline food that can help neutralize the body's acidity, especially helpful in the cases of large sugar consumption. They can be boiled in water and used as a tea, cold beverage, or salad dressing. The plums can be slivered and added to cooked vegetables, salads, and the center of rice balls. Umeboshi have a rare flavor that should be tried at least once!

UVA URSI   Also known as bearberry or mountain box, this bitter herb derived from the dried leaves of a trailing evergreen shrub (*Arctostaphylos uva ursi*) has long been used in cases of bladder inflammation and kidney disease. Uva ursi contains tannic acid, and should not be taken for more then two weeks in a succession or be used during pregnancy or by anyone suffering from kidney disorder. Uva ursi can be taken as a tea, a tincture, or in capsules.

V

VALERIAN TEA   Valerian root is one of the strongest of herbal sedatives. It induces sleep and is an excellent tranquilizer. The smell of this tea is nowadays considered rather unpleasant; but in sixteenth-century England, valerian root was appreciated as a fragrance and was placed among clothes as a perfume. In brewing valerian tea, never boil the root directly; pour boiling water over the root and steep like leaf tea. Some consider valerian to be more effective when soaked in cold water for 12 to 24 hours, strained, and downed without heating. However you brew it, do not take valerian tea for more than 14 days in a row. After a break of a week, another two-week stint can be embarked upon. In this manner, valerian's mildly addictive tendencies can be avoided while you enjoy its calming benefits. Valerian is also available in tincture form.

VANILLA BEAN   The vanilla bean is the long seedpod of a tropical orchid (imagine an orchid that is more valued for its seedpod than its flower!). After harvesting, it is dried and fermented and then develops the characteristic vanilla scent while crystals of vanillin form on the outside of the bean. The highest quality vanilla beans are 8 to 12 inches long, black in color, with vanillin crystals on the outside. Either inch-long pieces or the seeds scraped from the inside of the pod can be used for flavoring. A large vanilla bean will give you a lot of use if kept in an airtight container; slice or scrape it out as needed.

Many so-called vanilla extracts are made from synthetic vanillin, which is far cheaper than the real thing. As so little vanilla is called for to flavor any one recipe, it seems worthwhile to pay a little more for true and superbly flavored vanilla extract untainted by questionable additives.

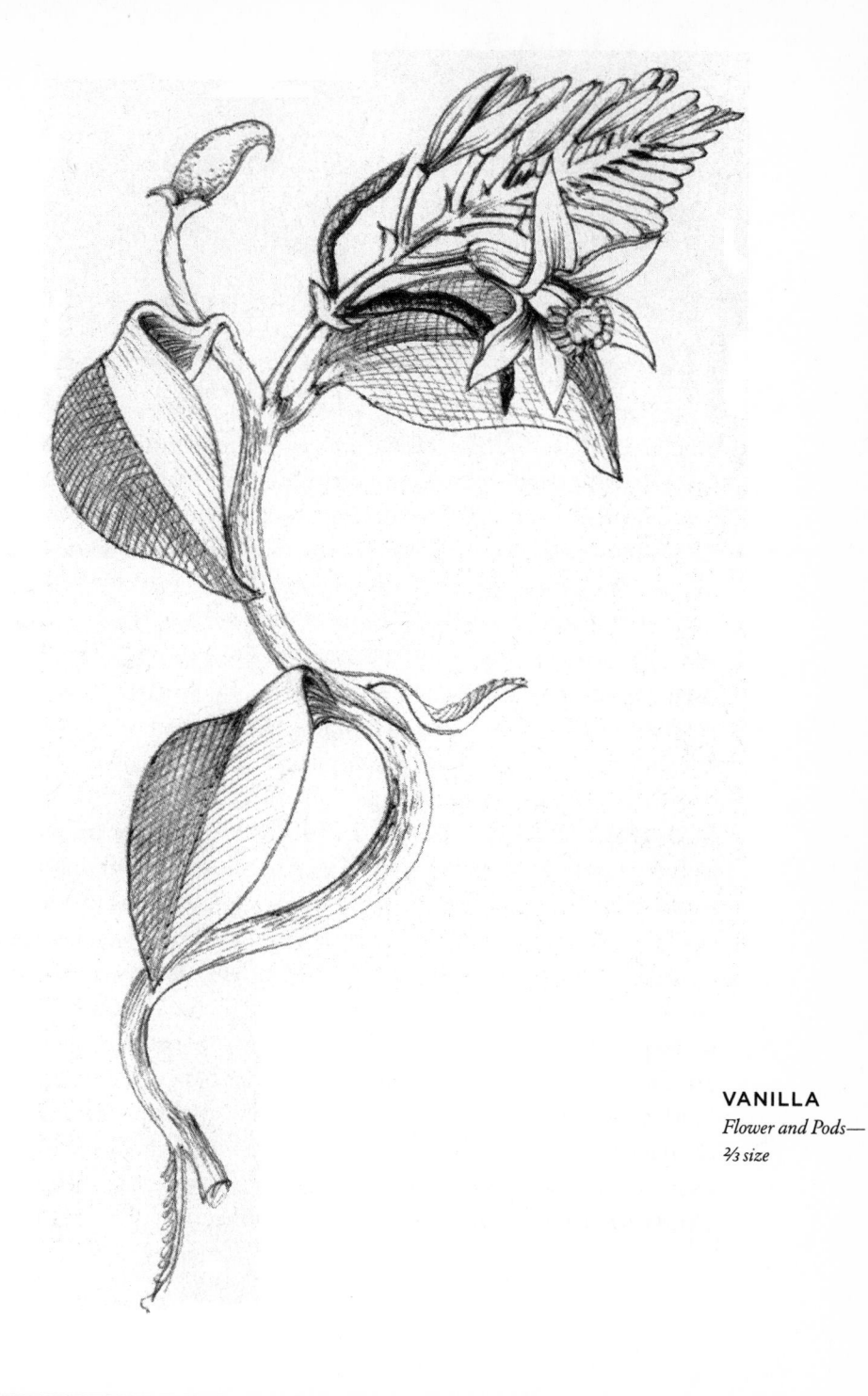

VANILLA
Flower and Pods—
⅔ size

VANILLA SUGAR

    1 (8-inch) vanilla bean

    1 cup sugar

- Chop the vanilla bean. Add it to the sugar, and grind with a mortar and pestle or in a blender. Place in a tightly closed jar for a week.
- Use measure for measure, whenever vanilla extract is called for.

VEGETABLES   See *Fruits and Vegetables, Fresh Organic.*

VERBASCUM   See *Mullein Blossom Tea.*

VINEGAR, APPLE CIDER   True vinegar is difficult to come by these days. That is, vinegar that is alive, a little cloudy with sediment, with mother (a viscid clump of yeast cells that develop in vinegar as it undergoes the natural process of acetous fermentation) resting at the bottom of the bottle. Cherish the mother—it can be used to make another batch of vinegar.

Most of the vinegar available commercially has been deadened by pasteurization, which results in vastly curtailed mineral content. Living apple cider vinegar made from whole apples is not only delicious in salads and cooking but also possesses many healthful attributes. It is very high in potassium, a most important mineral. A couple of teaspoons of vinegar taken in a glass of water with each meal is said to promote weight loss, prevent hardening of the arteries, waylay mild food poisoning, and ease migraines, high blood pressure, and dizziness. Use a teaspoon of apple cider vinegar to a glass of water as a gargle for sore throats; then swallow a sip of the gargle. Apply apple cider vinegar externally to ease bee stings, insect bites, poison ivy and poison oak, and burns. Use it as a hair rinse or in bath water to ease itchy skin. Add a touch of apple cider vinegar to meat marinades and broths; it draws the calcium out of the bones. Add it to the pickles you make; it helps them retain their natural food value.

The word "vinegar" comes from the French vinaigre, or sour wine. Good wine vinegar probably has many of the same healthful attributes as apple cider vinegar, but it is difficult to find unpasteurized wine vinegar in this country. You can make your own, however, by leaving a bottle of unpasteurized wine open and covered with a cloth for three to six months. Apple cider vinegar can be made in the same manner, using raw cider; the addition of a "mother" is not a requisite but hastens the acidifying process.

TROUT VINAIGRETTE

 ¼ cup raisins

 ¾ cup broth (or water)

 4 tablespoons olive oil

 ⅓ cup chopped onion

 1 clove garlic, chopped

 ¼ cup finely chopped celery

 ½ teaspoon dried sage (or 2 chopped fresh sage leaves)

 ½ teaspoon dried rosemary (or ¼ teaspoon chopped
  fresh rosemary)

 2 fresh trout (about 1 pound each)

 ¼ cup apple cider (or wine) vinegar

 1 teaspoon grated lemon peel

 1 teaspoon salt

 1 tablespoon unbleached white flour

 1 teaspoon soft butter

- Wash raisins and soak in the broth. In a frying pan large enough to hold the 2 trout (scraped and gutted, but with heads, tails, and fins intact), warm the olive oil and sauté the chopped onion, garlic, celery, sage, and rosemary until onion is transparent.

- Place the fish directly on top of the sauté, and sprinkle it with the vinegar and lemon peel. Add raisins, broth, and salt. Cover the pan and simmer over low heat for 10 minutes or until the fish flakes when gently probed with a fork. With the help of a spatula, gently lift the 2 trout out onto a prewarmed platter; pull off the top skin of the fish, up to the head.

- Blend the flour and soft butter with a fork. Stir it into the sauce, and let it simmer and thicken while you stir. Pour the sauce over the fish and serve.

- Provides joyous eating for two to four.

 COLESLAW

 5 cups shredded green cabbage

 5 cups shredded red cabbage

 2 cups shredded carrots

 ¼ cup apple cider vinegar

 ½ cup honey

 ½ cup mayonnaise (see recipe in book)

1 cup sour cream
1 tablespoon cinnamon
½ teaspoon ground ginger
Salt and pepper to taste

- Mix cabbages and carrots together. Mix all other ingredients together, then toss with cabbage and carrot mixture.
- Serves eight.

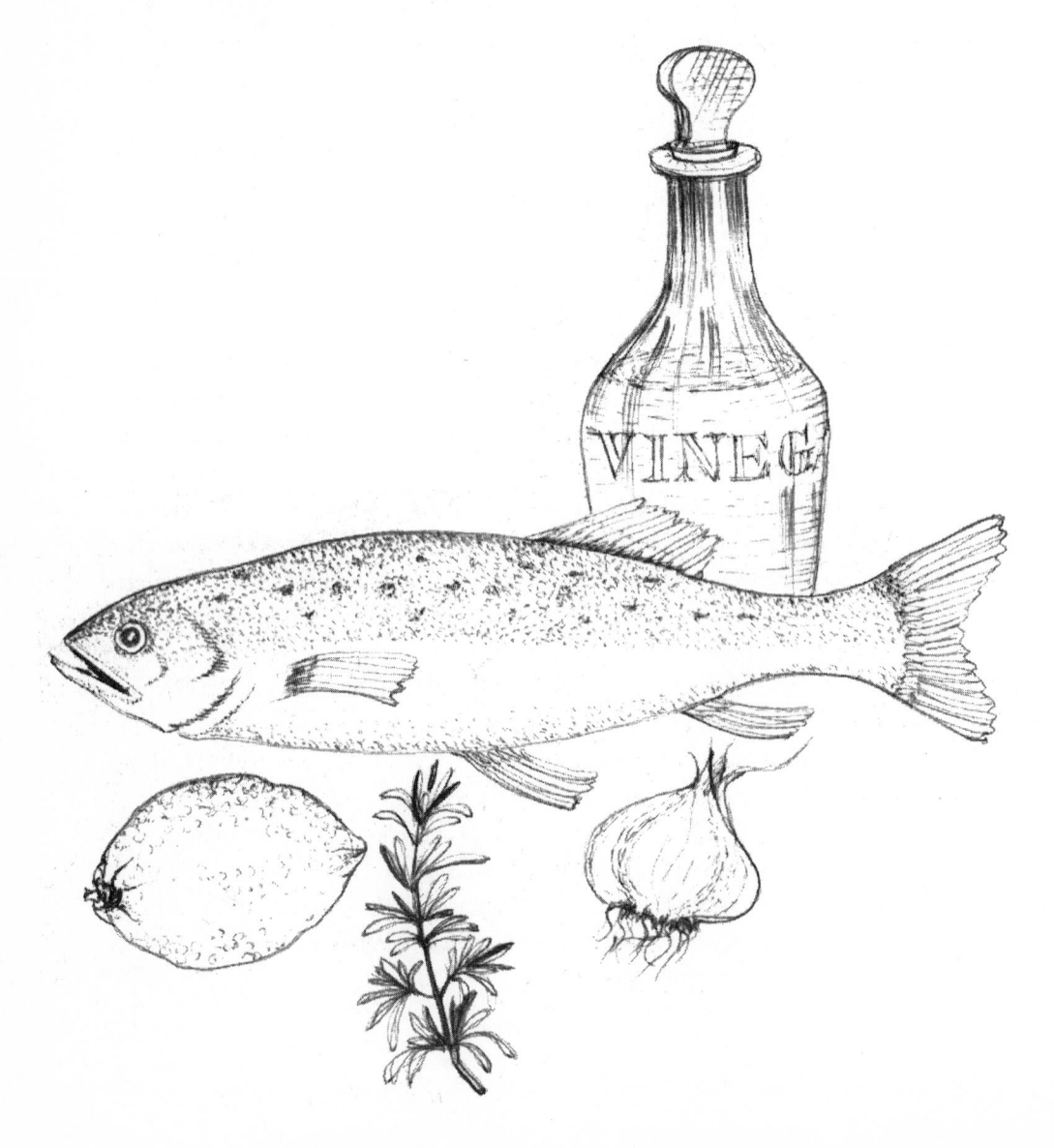

THE DICTIONARY OF WHOLESOME FOODS

VIOLET LEAF TEA The leaves of the violet are rich in vitamins A and C. Their tea (also known as pansy tea or heartsease—it gives ease to the heart, old tales say) is an excellent tonic, which is said to soothe headaches and should certainly help to chase away a cold. Steep 1 teaspoonful of chopped leaves in 2 cups boiling water for 10 minutes. Fresh violet blossoms and leaves are healthful and tasty—try chewing a few on a spring day.

VITAMINS Vitamins are organic substances that occur naturally in food and are essential to human health. Vitamins first began to be isolated and identified chemically at the beginning of the twentieth century, and as years have passed, ours has become an increasingly vitamin-conscious society.

Attitudes toward vitamins are enormously various and often at odds. Many claim that humans have, for thousands of years, obtained all the vitamins they need from their food, there is absolutely no reason why they should not continue to do so (even from standard refined supermarket fare), and that the business of vitamin supplements is unwarranted. Others feel that if one is careful to eat only unrefined foods, whole grains, and organically raised produce, extra vitamins become necessary only in times of illness and special stress. Still others embrace a daily regimen of vitamin supplements on the grounds that our food is so denatured that it cannot possibly supply all the necessary nutrients—and that this is accentuated by a sedentary way of life that cuts down on the amount of food we need, but not on the amount of vitamins our bodies require.

The debate over whether one should take synthetic or natural vitamins is also a large one. Many scientists assure us that because vitamins are in essence mere chemicals, they can be reproduced with exactitude in the laboratory. However, the makeup of a vitamin is not so simple. It can contain other nutritive elements and patterns that have not yet been isolated and that are essential to the proper absorption of the vitamin. Natural vitamins supply the needed nutrient in its natural food setting; such vitamins are therefore absorbed more completely and are also much less likely to produce the allergic reactions and toxic effects so common to synthetic vitamins. There are many companies that are anxious to cash in on the "natural" vitamin trend, and not all are to be trusted. Natural vitamins should be concentrates of actual food substances, with no artificial coloring or flavoring added; examine labels and when in doubt rely on well-known time-proven brands.

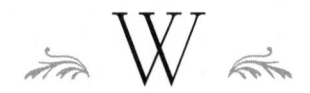

W

WAKAME   This seaweed is found in the cold turbulent waters of northern Japan and has a variety of uses. It may be added to soups or soaked for 15 minutes and then cooked by itself or with other vegetables. It can also be flipped over a burner flame until crisp, then crumbled and sprinkled over rice or noodles or served plain as a condiment. Wakame is rich in iodine and trace minerals.

WALNUT   There are many varieties of walnut trees that grow from China, through Europe, to North America. Their wood is highly valued for carpentry, and their leaves and nutshells for a black dye. Their kernels yield an oil used by both cooks and artists. The delicious kernels produced by most walnut trees are high in incomplete protein, unsaturated fatty acids, B vitamins, potassium, phosphorus, trace minerals, and omega-3s. Black walnuts, which are indigenous to North America, are tedious to shell but contain more nutrients than English walnuts. Two or three walnuts a day are said to alleviate bursitis symptoms.

Commercially treated walnuts are often bleached with lye to produce uniformity of color and are gassed to make shelling easier. Try to obtain these nuts in their pristine state.

WALNUT OIL   This highly unsaturated oil is cold pressed from dried walnuts. Walnut oil has a definite nutty flavor and is not appreciated by everyone; so try it first in small amounts, in salads or cooking.

WASABI   Traditionally served with raw fish, sushi, or Japanese soba dishes, the pale green wasabi rhizome is best when grated and served fresh. Most commercial wasabi powders on the market are not made from wasabi at all, but from a mixture of horseradish, mustard, and food coloring. When fresh wasabi root

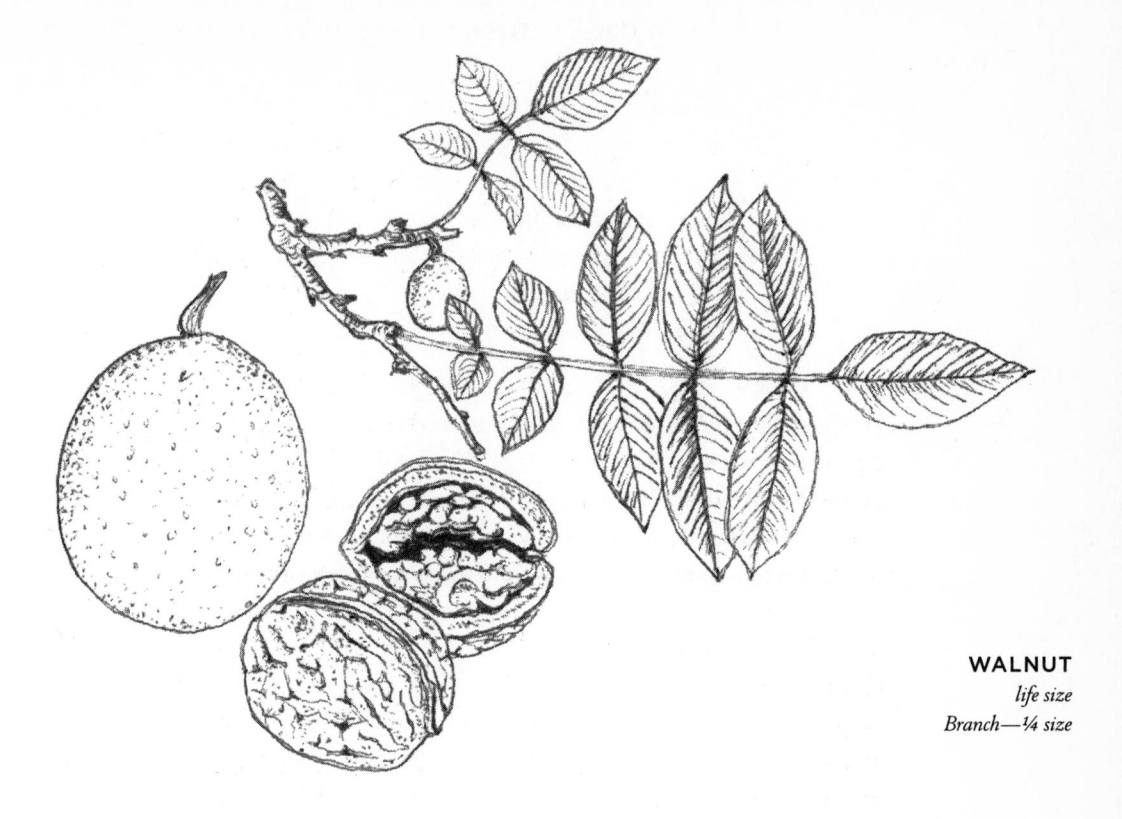

WALNUT
life size
Branch—¼ size

is unavailable, be sure to seek out wasabi paste or powder that has been made from the real thing. Avoid vibrantly green imitations.

WATERMELON TEA   Crush watermelon seeds in a blender or mortar and steep 1 tablespoonful in 2 cups boiling water for 30 minutes. Strain this brew and you will have a tea that is said to be helpful for kidney problems and high blood pressure.

WHEAT BERRIES   Also referred to as groats, wheat berries are whole wheat kernels that have not been milled, polished, or heat-treated. Missing only their inedible outer husk, wheat berries, with their robust, nutty flavor, are nutritionally intact and make magnificent pilafs, casseroles, soups, and yeast breads. Wheat berries take about an hour to cook if soaked for eight hours prior to cooking, so some planning ahead is necessary.

BUFFET WHEAT BERRY AND BARLEY PILAF

1 cup wheat berries

1 cup barley

9 tablespoons butter

2 large onions, sliced

2 tablespoons fresh thyme

2/3 cup dry toasted almonds, cut into matchsticks

1/2 cup chopped parsley

Salt and pepper

- Cook wheat berries in salted water to cover for 2 hours or until tender. Drain. Cook barley in 3 cups salted water for 45 minutes or until tender. Drain. (Do not cook together.)
- Melt 6 tablespoons butter in a frying pan. Add onions. Cook over medium heat, stirring until caramelized, about 25–30 minutes. Mix barley, wheat berries, thyme, onion, 3 tablespoons butter, nuts, and 1/3 cup parsley. Add salt and pepper. Mix well in a large bowl and garnish with remaining parsley.
- Serves twelve.

WHEAT, CRACKED   The cracked grain of wheat—each kernel is split into about 4 or 5 pieces—has all the nutritional value found in whole grain wheat, plus a convenience factor. It is short cooking; as a cereal or a rice substitute, it can be whipped up in about 10 minutes, using 1 cup grain to 2 cups water or milk or broth. It can also be eaten without cooking if soaked in water to cover overnight, making it a good item for camping trips. And it can be used as a binder in meat loaves and hamburgers, and in soups and stews. See also *Wheat Grain*.

WHEAT GERM, RAW   The germ is the embryo of the wheat kernel, its veritable life force. It is one of the richest known sources of vitamins E and B_1, and contains iron and protein. Unfortunately it is considered expendable—even undesirable—by large wheat processors, and its healthful presence is not to be found in the refined flour and cereals that crowd supermarket shelves. The vitamin E–rich oil of the wheat germ soon becomes rancid unless refrigerated, so it has no place in the denatured flours that are meant to last forever in vast storage bins and on market shelves. The only advantage to this situation is that there is a lot of plain pure wheat germ to be had, and its healthful presence should be felt in every kitchen.

Raw wheat germ must be kept refrigerated in a tightly covered container. It can be cooked in milk as a breakfast cereal or mixed with other cereals to strengthen their nutritional value. It can be added to bread dough, but should be simmered in milk or lightly toasted first. If you like the taste of raw wheat germ, sprinkle it over yogurt and cottage cheese dishes. If toasted wheat germ is preferred, roast it lightly in a heavy skillet on top of the stove or bake it in the oven (see *Wheat Germ, Toasted*).

BAKED STUFFED ZUCCHINI

6 medium-large (8–10 inches long) zucchini

8 tablespoons olive oil

4 medium-size onions, chopped

3 cloves garlic, chopped

$\frac{1}{4}$ cup fresh parsley, chopped (or 2 tablespoons dry)

$\frac{1}{2}$ teaspoon fresh oregano, chopped (or $\frac{1}{4}$ teaspoon dry)

$\frac{1}{2}$ teaspoon fresh basil, chopped (or $\frac{1}{4}$ teaspoon dry)

$1\frac{1}{2}$ teaspoons salt

$\frac{1}{4}$ teaspoon freshly ground black pepper

6 tablespoons grated Parmesan cheese

$\frac{1}{4}$ cup whole wheat bread crumbs (bread crumbs can be made in blender or crumbled finely by hand)

TOPPING:

$\frac{1}{2}$ cup whole wheat bread crumbs

$\frac{1}{4}$ cup wheat germ, raw or toasted

$\frac{2}{3}$ cup Parmesan cheese, grated

$\frac{1}{2}$ teaspoon salt

$\frac{1}{8}$ teaspoon freshly ground black pepper

$\frac{1}{4}$ teaspoon paprika

- Slice the zucchini in half lengthwise and scoop out the insides, leaving walls about ¼ inch thick. Place the zucchini shells in an oiled baking dish and bake at 300 degrees for 30 minutes.

- Meanwhile, sauté in oil the onions, garlic, and coarsely chopped zucchini pulp until all are tender. Then add parsley, oregano, basil, salt, and pepper and simmer covered for 5 minutes. Remove from stove, mash with a fork, and add Parmesan cheese and bread crumbs. In a separate bowl mix together the topping ingredients.

- Fill the baked zucchini shells with the pulp mixture and cover with topping. Bake at 300 degrees for 30 minutes.
- Serves four to five.
- *Note:* If there is not enough filling for all the zucchini shells, save the shells to put in soup.

WHEAT GERM, TOASTED Toasted wheat germ has a crisp nutlike flavor that many people savor by the spoonful alone. But it has a myriad of other uses as well. Use it as a cereal or on other cereal; use it along with or instead of bread crumbs for topping casseroles or breading meats and fish; add it to cookies and breads, use it in crumb toppings for desserts.

Wheat germ loses some of its health value when it is toasted, but the loss can be kept to a minimum if you toast it yourself. Commercially prepared toasted wheat germ (and this includes some health food brands) often has had its vitamin E–rich oil removed. See also *Wheat Germ, Raw.*

TOASTED WHEAT GERM

2 cups raw wheat germ

- Put the wheat germ in a heavy skillet over medium-high heat and roast, stirring, until a toasted aroma arises and the germ is lightly browned. Cool and store in a tightly covered container.
- Or spread the raw wheat germ on a baking sheet and roast in a preheated 300-degree oven for 10–15 minutes or until lightly browned. Cool and store in a tightly covered container.
- Toasted wheat germ does not require refrigeration unless the weather is particularly hot, or you plan to keep it for over a month.

WHEAT GERM FLOUR Wheat germ flour is made by finely grinding raw wheat germ. It can be added to breads, cakes, and cookies, and lends a finer texture to baked goods than does the whole wheat germ. This highly nutritious item is very perishable and should be kept refrigerated.

WHEAT GRAIN Whole wheat grains are rich in magnesium, iron, phosphorus, vitamins B and E, carbohydrates, and numerous trace minerals. By the time the food industry has finished processing this nutritious grain for flours and cereals, there is little left but carbohydrates—and a few synthetic nutrients thrown in for good measure.

Whole grains of wheat can be used for cereal, but they take a lot of cooking. Usually wheat grain is purchased by those who grind their own flour. The taste and nutritional value of freshly ground flour are unsurpassable. So if you are really into making your own bread, consider investing in a small stone grinding mill (expensive) or a hand grinder (less expensive). Wheat grain preserves itself with its own hard covering, so problems of refrigeration are eliminated.

WHEAT GRASS   Ever wonder why so many juice bars sport flats of grass right next to the pile of carrots? Well, wonder no further. Yes, it is grass, and yes, it is for making juice, and yes again, people actually drink it. High in vitamins A, B, C, and E as well as amino acids, this is one grass that isn't just for bovines. With its high chlorophyll content, many believe wheat grass to be a veritable fountain of health, beneficial in the prevention and curing of cancer, improving digestion, neutralizing toxins in the body, and providing a caffeine-free energy boost on the spot.

Wheat grass flats can be nurtured easily at home but necessitate a special, and quite costly, wheat grass juicer. Many aficionados, however, deem it worth the expense to have fresh wheat grass juice on hand, and so invest in both a wheat grass juicer and a vegetable juicer. For those who do not mind the sweet but distinctly grassy taste of wheat grass, drink one or two ounces a day straight from the glass, and make sure it's fresh from the press, as wheat grass very quickly loses its nutrients. However, if drinking wheat grass seems reminiscent of inhaling a mouthful of lawn clippings, try mixing wheat grass with other vegetable juices—especially carrot—as a way of mellowing out what can be an overwhelming taste sensation.

WHEAT GRITS   The whole wheat kernel is coarsely ground to obtain wheat grits. Grits are similar to cracked wheat but finer in grind. Add to bread, cereal, meat loaf, and hamburgers. See also *Wheat Grain*.

WHEY POWDER   During cheese making, the milk separates into curds and whey. The whey is watery, somewhat tart, and very high in B vitamins. Whey is available in dried form and is a nutritious addition to blended beverages. Like other cultured milk products, it fosters the growth of necessary bacteria in the intestinal tract and aids digestion. Whey powder can also be added to baked goods.

WHITE FLOUR, UNBLEACHED   Unbleached white flour provides a halfway point where those who have turned their backs on refined foods can rest their senses before climbing on to more exclusive use of whole grains. This flour certainly is not the epitome of healthfulness, but it is a far sight better than the bleached white nonsense that is found in our supermarkets. It has had most of the bran and germ removed, but has not been bleached with harmful chlorides and is often grown organically. It is very useful if your tastes lean toward flaky French pastries, light airy cakes, and Italian loaves of bread. It can be substituted in any recipe calling for white flour. If you would like to gradually wean your family (and possibly yourself) away from lily-white bread, start by using unbleached white flour mixed with ordinary dead white flour; then move on to just unbleached white; then start adding whole wheat flour by the half cupful. Chances are the delicious taste of whole grains will creep up on everyone until it is accepted as the norm.

WHOLE WHEAT BREAD FLOUR   Whole wheat flour has made a comeback. And it is about time. How tasteless and chemically manipulated white flour could have eclipsed the rare goodness of whole grain flour is somewhat mysterious; perhaps in the deluge of easily available cheap white flour, people simply forgot what *true* flour can actually do to a loaf of bread.

In making whole wheat flour, the entire kernel of wheat has traditionally been stone ground between enormous round buhr stones. The molecular structure of the wheat kernel remains intact and the flour does not reach high temperatures, thus ensuring the preservation of essential nutrients that are destroyed by commercial milling techniques. Another method of grinding—pneumatic milling—has laid claim to the same nutritional results as traditional stone grinding.

True whole wheat flour is not available in ordinary commercial stores. What is marketed as "whole wheat flour" is usually bleached flour with some bran added to give a whole grain "look." The germ, the most essential ingredient, is entirely missing because the germ possesses an oil that in time becomes rancid without refrigeration, and its presence is therefore not conducive to the endless shelf life required of commercial foodstuffs.

When buying whole wheat flour from a health food store, be careful to pick a brand that seems to have a high sales turnover. The longer flour sits on the shelf, the more nutrients it loses. And do not buy more than enough to last a month; it is best to buy small quantities frequently, to ensure that the flour does not get stale on your shelf. Of course the ideal way to have whole grain flour is to grind it yourself as you need it. The fresher the grind, the better the taste and the higher the nutritional value.

Whole wheat flour is an excellent source of B vitamins and also contains magnesium, potassium, iron, vitamin E, and protein. Most of these nutrients are concentrated in the bran and germ of the wheat. When they are removed by refining, no amount of "enrichment" with synthetic nutrients is going to restore the natural healthful state of the flour.

Whole wheat flour can be made from hard (spring) wheat or soft (winter wheat). Hard wheat contains more protein, in the form of gluten, and makes the best bread. Soft wheat is used for all-purpose and pastry flour, although it can be blended with hard wheat to make bread.

WHOLE WHEAT BREAD

    1 tablespoon dry yeast (or 2 ounces compressed)
    ½ cup lukewarm water
    3 tablespoons pressed oil (soy is good)
    2 tablespoons honey or molasses
    2 cups water or milk (lukewarm)
    1½ teaspoons salt
    5½ cups whole wheat flour

- Dissolve yeast in ½ cup lukewarm water until it foams. Add oil and honey and stir well. Add 2 cups lukewarm water or milk; then sift in salt and half of the flour. Stir very well. Add more flour until the dough is too stiff to stir. Put it onto a floured board and knead in the remainder of the flour, using more flour if necessary, until the dough is no longer sticky and forms a smooth, neat ball. This should take 5–10 minutes of kneading.

- Place the ball of dough in a large lightly oiled bowl, cover with a tea towel, and place in a warm spot. Let it rise until double in bulk (about 1 hour). Punch down the dough, kneading lightly to express all the air. Shape into 2 loaves and place in oiled bread pans. Set the oven at 375 degrees. Let the loaves rise (again covered, in a warm spot) until dough just reaches the top of the pans. Put in the oven and bake for 10 minutes. Then turn the oven down to 350 degrees and continue baking for 40 minutes or until loaves are browned and sound hollow when tapped. Remove from the oven and the pans, and cool the loaves on their sides on a rack.

- Makes 2 medium-size loaves.

- *Notes on bread making:* Have all ingredients at room temperature before starting. Measure oil first, and then use the same spoon for the honey—the honey will then slip right off with no sticky mess. The amount of flour to use is always variable, depending on the type of flour, the weather, the altitude, etc.; develop a "feel" for what is right. Stir and knead vigorously; this spreads the yeast and develops the gluten, making light and evenly rising loaves. Try using coffee cans for bread pans—they make a nice shape for sandwiches; but take care to fill them only half full with dough. Cool loaves on their sides on a cake rack; this will help keep them from being bottom heavy.

WHOLE WHEAT PASTRY FLOUR   Whole wheat pastry flour is made from soft winter wheat. Because it is lower in gluten than flour derived from hard wheat, it makes cakes and pastries that are tender and finely textured. If you are unable to locate whole wheat pastry flour, sift regular whole wheat flour a half-dozen times through a fine mesh sifter, reserving the bran that will not pass through for bread making. Also, make certain not to overbeat the batter (this will keep the gluten from developing and will give a tenderer cake), and add 1 teaspoon more baking powder than is called for in the recipe. Whole wheat pastry flour can be substituted cup for cup in any recipe calling for white pastry or all-purpose flour. For a lighter cake, add ½ to 1 teaspoon more baking powder. Whole wheat pastry flour can be mixed with regular whole wheat flour to make bread, but if used alone the result will be a very heavy loaf because of the lower gluten of this flour.

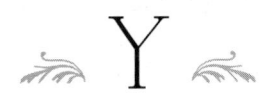

Y

YARROW TEA This familiar roadside herb (*Achillea millefolia*) is also known as *milfoil* because of the many fine divisions of its leaves. Although yarrow was long ago said to ward off evil spirits, today it is primarily used to stimulate the appetite and to alleviate colitis symptoms. Tea can be made from either the fresh or dried leaves and flowers. It is astringent and can be used externally to treat oily skin and hair.

YEAST, BAKING Baking yeast is a living plant. Given a warm and moist environment, the yeast cells start to grow, and it is this growth that causes bread to rise. If the temperature is too cold or too hot, the yeast will not function; this is why all ingredients involved in bread making must be lukewarm or at room temperature, why rising must take place in a warm spot, and why the loaf stops rising soon after being placed in a hot oven.

Yeast is available commercially in two forms: dry or compressed. Dry yeast will keep for about six months. Compressed yeast is extremely perishable and should be used within a week, although it can be frozen successfully for longer periods of time. When its light gray color turns to brown, it is too old to use.

YEAST, BREWER'S See *Brewer's Yeast.*

YERBA MATÉ TEA This tea is the national drink in many parts of South America and is made from the dried leaves of the maté evergreen tree. It has been used since time immemorial by the South American Indians (maté is the Inca word for the gourdlike vessel originally used to hold the beverage) and quickly picked up by the invading Portuguese and Spaniards, who added "yerba" (meaning "herb") to its name. It is a stimulating and nourishing tea and is preferred by some to black tea because of its almost nonexistent caffeine content, its naturally stimulating effect, and its vitamin and mineral content. Use 1 tablespoon maté to 2 cups boiling water; steep for 3 to 5 minutes, strain, and serve; or even better, enjoy your maté using the traditional maté cup and bombilla, the straw through which the maté is meant to be drunk. Fill the maté gourd or cup three-quarters of the way full with maté, and then cover with hot water and drink. The maté is meant to be repeatedly covered with hot water and enjoyed until little flavor remains in the leaves, at which point they can be dumped and replenished with new. Recent reports claim that yerba mate may have carcinogenic properties and that, like coffee, it should not be consumed in excessive amounts.

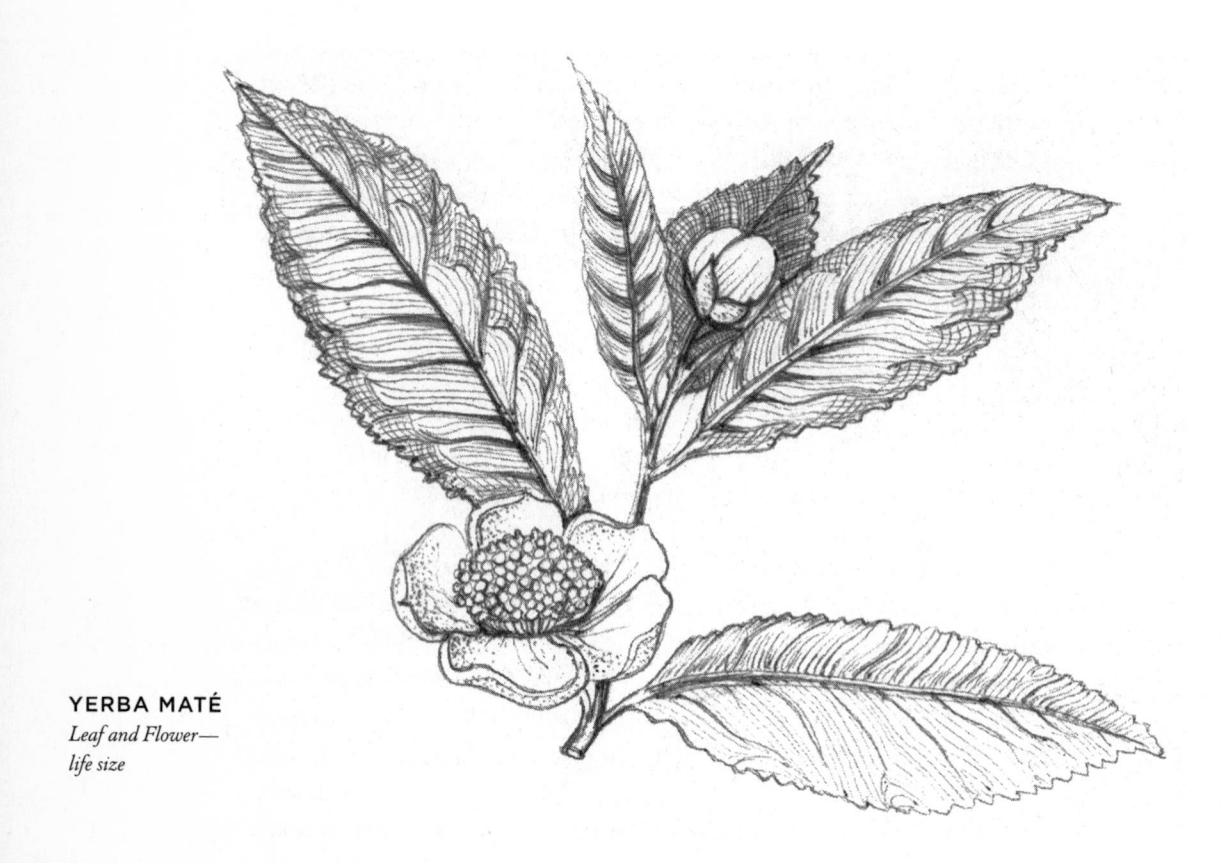

YERBA MATÉ
*Leaf and Flower—
life size*

YERBA SANTA TEA　This "holy herb" tea grows in California and was long used by the West Coast Native Americans to alleviate bronchial problems such as asthma, laryngitis, and hay fever. Its aromatic flavor and medicinal effects are still appreciated by herbal tea drinkers.

YOGURT   Yogurt is a cultured milk product that is custardlike in consistency and sour in taste. It has been enjoyed for thousands of years by Eastern Europeans and has come into its own in this country. Its health benefits are so numerous as to be almost legendary. This is the item that is said to produce all the centenarians in far-off Hunza (Pakistan) villages. There is certainly no doubt that yogurt is very rich in B vitamins and calcium, and because of its high count of healthy bacteria, it is extremely useful in conditioning the intestinal tract. It soothes stomach ulcers, regulates the bowels in cases of constipation or diarrhea, is far easier to digest than milk, and helps repair the damage that antibiotics wreak upon the intestinal tract. It is also a delicious and extremely versatile food that can be used for breakfast, lunch, or dinner, as dessert, beverage, sauce, soup, or garnish.

Commercial yogurts may contain jelling agents, artificial flavoring and coloring, preservatives, and lots of sugar. Particularly avoid the flavored types; they are easily made at home using more healthful ingredients. The yogurt carried in health food stores should be dependably additive free. But you can save yourself a lot of money by making your own yogurt at home. It is very simple to do, and especially delicious to taste.

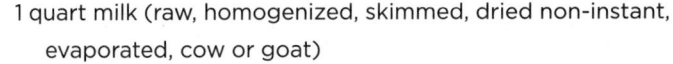

HOMEMADE YOGURT

> 1 quart milk (raw, homogenized, skimmed, dried non-instant, evaporated, cow or goat)
>
> 3 tablespoons non-instant dried milk (optional, gives a firmer yogurt)
>
> 3 tablespoons unflavored yogurt (or a dry yogurt culture)
>
> Jars with tops

Put the milk into a heavy pot and place over low heat. If you choose to add the dry milk, mix it into a smooth paste with a small amount of milk and stir it into the rest of the milk. Scald the milk; it should be steaming hot but not boiling. Remove from heat and let it cool to about 110 degrees (lukewarm) on a candy thermometer or until you can hold your finger in it for 10 seconds without burning. Cooling can be hastened by setting the pot of hot milk in a sink of cold water. When the milk has cooled to the proper temperature, mix in the fresh yogurt or yogurt culture, making sure there are no lumps. Then ladle the mixture into clean jars and cap them.

The point now is to keep the yogurt at about 110 degrees for 3–8 hours. And here is where variety of approach creeps in. You can put the yogurt-filled bottles in a heavy pot with a few inches of warm water in it and set it over a pilot light, on a warm (*not hot*) radiator, or in an oven that is warmed by a pilot light or turned on periodically to keep the atmosphere at about 110 degrees. Or put the jars in an electric frying pan shallowly filled with water and keep it at the lowest heat adjustment. In all cases, check the water temperature occasionally (with a thermometer or the 10-count finger test). If it is too cold the yogurt will not jell, and if it is too hot the yogurt bacteria will die and the milk will curdle.

Yogurt made with fresh yogurt as culture usually takes 3 to 5 hours to jell; made with dried yogurt culture, it takes longer—up to 8 hours. When the yogurt is ready (test by tipping a jar slightly or inserting a knife to test its firmness—the yogurt will become firmer with refrigeration), remove from the water and refrigerate. Enjoy yogurt plain, or sweetened with honey or maple syrup. Flavor it with jam or fresh fruit. For vanilla or coffee flavor, add vanilla extract or instant coffee with a little honey.

YOGURT BREAKFAST

> 2 cups yogurt
> 2 oranges, peeled and chopped
> 1 apple, chopped
> ½ cup nuts, chopped
> 3 tablespoons raisins
> 6 tablespoons wheat germ
> 2 tablespoons honey

Mix all ingredients together and serve immediately.

Serves three to four.

RAITA

> 2 cups plain yogurt
> 1 small cucumber, chopped
> ½ cup fresh mint, chopped
> 1 tablespoon cumin
> Salt and pepper to taste

Mix all ingredients together at least 2 hours before serving. (May be made the night before.) Chill until you wish to serve. Garnish with extra mint leaves. Wonderful served with any curry dish as a condiment.

Serves four.

CURRIED EGGPLANT WITH YOGURT

1 medium-size (1–2 pounds) eggplant

1 medium onion, chopped

5 tablespoons vegetable oil (preferably pressed oil)

2 teaspoons ground coriander

2–3 teaspoons curry powder

1 tablespoon tomato paste

1 teaspoon salt

1 cup yogurt

- Slash the eggplant in several places with a knife, and bake in a 400-degree oven for 25–35 minutes or until tender. Cool the eggplant; then peel and chop it coarsely.

- In a skillet, sauté the chopped onion in the oil. When it is tender but not brown, add the coriander and curry powder (using a lesser amount if your curry powder is very strong, and more if it is mild), and cook for a couple of minutes. Stir in the tomato paste. Then add the eggplant and salt and simmer, while stirring, for 5 minutes. Spoon into a bowl, stir in the yogurt, and refrigerate.

- Serve chilled as an appetizer or as an accompaniment to a main course of curry.

- Serves four to six.

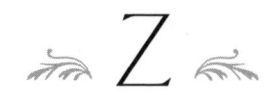

Z

ZA'ATAR   This aromatic seasoning from the Middle East is a finely ground spice blend of sesame seeds, thyme, marjoram, and sumac. Za'atar can be made at home or purchased at specialty stores. Za'atar can be mixed with olive oil to form a paste and basted onto lamb or chicken, or drizzled over hot pita bread. Useful as a seasoning for meats, salads, or vegetables, za'atar is sure to add an exotic Middle Eastern flair to any dish.

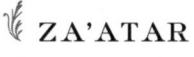 **ZA'ATAR**

  ½ cup sesame seeds, toasted, and coarsely ground
  ¼ cup sumac
  2 teaspoons ground oregano
  2 teaspoons savory
  2 teaspoons ground marjoram
  4 tablespoons ground thyme
  1 teaspoon salt, or to taste

Mix together all ingredients and then grind, or crush using a pestle or a spice mill, should you have one, or place the spice mixture in a zip lock plastic bag and crush with a rolling pin. Store your za'atar in an airtight container.

RECIPE INDEX

THE DICTIONARY OF WHOLESOME FOODS